FDG-PET/CT Imaging in Infectious and Inflammatory Disorders

Editors

LARS CHRISTIAN GORMSEN
SØREN HESS

PET CLINICS

www.pet.theclinics.com

Consulting Editor
ABASS ALAVI

April 2020 • Volume 15 • Number 2

ELSEVIER

1600 John F. Kennedy Boulevard • Suite 1800 • Philadelphia, Pennsylvania, 19103-2899

http://www.pet.theclinics.com

PET CLINICS Volume 15, Number 2
April 2020 ISSN 1556-8598, ISBN-13: 978-0-323-71082-4

Editor: John Vassallo (j.vassallo@elsevier.com)
Developmental Editor: Casey Potter

PET Clinics (ISSN 1556-8598) is published quarterly by Elsevier Inc., 360 Park Avenue South, New York, NY 10010-1710. Months of issue are January, April, July, and October. Periodicals postage paid at New York, NY, and additional mailing offices. Subscription prices per year are $247.00 (US individuals), $422.00 (US institutions), $100.00 (US students), $279.00 (Canadian individuals), $475.00 (Canadian institutions), $100.00 (Canadian students), $275.00 (foreign individuals), $475.00 (foreign institutions), and $140.00 (foreign students). To receive student and resident rate, orders must be accompanied by name of affiliated institution, date of term, and the signature of program/residency coordinator on institution letterhead. Orders will be billed at individual rate until proof of status is received. Foreign air speed delivery is included in all Clinics subscription prices. All prices are subject to change without notice. POSTMASTER: Send address changes to PET Clinics, Elsevier Health Sciences Division, Subscription Customer Service, 3251 Riverport Lane, Maryland Heights, MO 63043. **Customer Service: 1-800-654-2452 (U.S. and Canada); 314-447-8871 (outside U.S. and Canada). Fax: 314-447-8029. E-mail: journalscustomerservice-usa@elsevier.com (for print support); journalsonlinesupport-usa@elsevier.com (for online support).**

Reprints. For copies of 100 or more of articles in this publication, please contact the Commercial Reprints Department, Elsevier Inc., 360 Park Avenue South, New York, NY 10010-1710. Tel.: 212-633-3874; Fax: 212-633-3820; E-mail: reprints@elsevier.com.

PET Clinics is covered in MEDLINE/PubMed (Index Medicus).

Contributors

CONSULTING EDITOR

ABASS ALAVI, MD, MD (Hon), PhD (Hon), DSc (Hon)
Professor of Radiology, Division of Nuclear Medicine, Department of Radiology,
Hospital of the University of Pennsylvania, University of Pennsylvania Perelman School of Medicine, Philadelphia, Pennsylvania, USA

EDITORS

LARS CHRISTIAN GORMSEN, MD, PhD
Senior Chief Physician, Associate Professor, Head of Research, Department of Nuclear Medicine and PET Centre, Aarhus University Hospital, Department of Clinical Medicine, Aarhus University, Aarhus, Denmark
(Nuclear Medicine and PET), Department of Radiology and Nuclear Medicine, Hospital of Southwest Jutland, Esbjerg, Denmark; Faculty of Health Sciences, Department of Regional Health Research, University of Southern Denmark, Odense, Denmark

SØREN HESS, MD
Senior Consultant, Associate Professor, Head of Research (Imaging), Head of Section

AUTHORS

MINA AL NAJAFI, MD
National Heart, Lung, Blood Institute, National Institutes of Health, Bethesda, Maryland, USA

ABASS ALAVI, MD, MD (Hon), PhD (Hon), DSc (Hon)
Professor of Radiology, Division of Nuclear Medicine, Department of Radiology, Hospital of the University of Pennsylvania, University of Pennsylvania Perelman School of Medicine, Philadelphia, Pennsylvania, USA

SANDIP BASU, MBBS (Hons), DRM, DNB
Radiation Medicine Centre (BARC), Tata Memorial Hospital Annexe, Homi Bhabha National Institute, Mumbai, India

ALBRECHT BETRAINS, MD
Department of General Internal Medicine, University Hospital Gasthuisberg, Leuven, Belgium

GREGORY BISSON, MD, MSCE
Center for Clinical Epidemiology and Biostatistics, University of Pennsylvania, Philadelphia, USA

DANIEL BLOCKMANS, MD, PhD
Department of General Internal Medicine, University Hospital Gasthuisberg, Leuven, Belgium

JACOB BRODER BRODERSEN, MD
Department of Gastroenterology, Hospital of Southwest Jutland, Esbjerg, Denmark

BANGKIM CHANDRA KHANGEMBAM, MD, FANMB
Assistant Professor, Department of Nuclear Medicine, All India Institute of Medical Sciences, New Delhi, India

VIPLAV DEOGAONKAR, MBBS
Department of Radiology, Hospital of University of Pennsylvania, Philadelphia, Pennsylvania, USA

AMIT K. DEY, MD
National Heart, Lung, Blood Institute, National Institutes of Health, Bethesda, Maryland, USA

LARS CHRISTIAN GORMSEN, MD, PhD
Senior Chief Physician, Associate Professor, Head of Research, Department of Nuclear Medicine and PET Centre, Aarhus University Hospital, Department of Clinical Medicine, Aarhus University, Aarhus, Denmark

SØREN HESS, MD
Senior Consultant, Associate Professor, Head of Research (Imaging), Head of Section (Nuclear Medicine and PET), Department of Radiology and Nuclear Medicine, Hospital of Southwest Jutland, Esbjerg, Denmark; Department of Regional Health Research, University of Southern Denmark, Odense, Denmark

ASHWINI KALSHETTY, DNB
Radiation Medicine Centre (BARC), Tata Memorial Hospital Annexe, Homi Bhabha National Institute, Mumbai, India

MALTE KIRCHER, MD
Department of Nuclear Medicine, University Hospital Augsburg, Würzburg, Germany

RAKESH KUMAR, MD, PhD
Professor and Head, Diagnostic Nuclear Medicine Division, All India Institute of Medical Sciences, New Delhi, India

ROBERT M. KWEE, MD, PhD
Department of Radiology, Zuyderland Medical Center, Heerlen/Sittard/Geleen, The Netherlands

THOMAS C. KWEE, MD, PhD
Department of Radiology, Nuclear Medicine and Molecular Imaging, University Medical Center Groningen, University of Groningen, Groningen, The Netherlands

CONSTANTIN LAPA, MD
Department of Nuclear Medicine, University Hospital Augsburg, Würzburg, Germany

NEHAL N. MEHTA, MD, MSCE
Chief, Section of Inflammation and Cardiometabolic Diseases, National Heart, Lung and Blood Institute, Clinical Research Center, Bethesda, Maryland, USA

BERIT DALSGAARD NIELSEN, MD, PhD
Department of Rheumatology, Aarhus University Hospital, Aarhus, Aarhus N, Denmark; Department of Clinical Medicine, Aarhus University, Department of Nuclear Medicine and PET Centre, Aarhus University Hospital, Aarhus, Denmark

AARTHI S. REDDY, BS
National Heart, Lung, Blood Institute, National Institutes of Health, Bethesda, Maryland, USA

ASBJØRN MATHIAS SCHOLTENS, MD
Meander Medical Center, Nuclear Medicine Physician, Nuclear Medicine, Amersfoort, The Netherlands

SIAVASH MEHDIZADEH SERAJ, MD
Department of Radiology, Hospital of University of Pennsylvania, Philadelphia, Pennsylvania, USA

DOMINGO E. UCEDA, BS
National Heart, Lung, Blood Institute, National Institutes of Health, Bethesda, Maryland, USA

MBOYO-DI-TAMBA VANGU, MD, MMed
Department of Nuclear Medicine, University of Johannesburg, Auckland Park, South Africa

Contents

Several factors that influence physiologic 18F-fluorodeoxyglucose (FDG) uptake and general FDG distribution may affect PET/CT imaging in infection and inflammation. The general impact of hyperglycemia on the diagnostic performance of FDG-PET/CT is probably less in infection/inflammation than in malignancy. Patient preparation may reduce physiologic FDG uptake, but recommendations are less established than in malignancy. Local implementation of various patient preparatory measures should reflect the specific patient population and indications. This article outlines some of the challenges with physiologic FDG distribution, focusing on infectious and inflammatory diseases, and potential countermeasures and patient preparation to limit physiologic uptake before scan.

18F-Fluorodeoxyglucose (FDG) PET/computed tomography (CT) is a highly accurate diagnostic tool for large vessel vasculitis (LVV) and is one of the recommended imaging modalities for confirmation of the diagnosis. This article focuses on the role of FDG-PET/CT in LVV diagnosis and disease monitoring, mainly focusing on giant cell arteritis; in particular, the diagnostic accuracy, diagnostic criteria, the potential pitfalls in the interpretation of large vessel FDG uptake, and the clinical indication compared with other imaging modalities are discussed.

The increasing implementation of advanced imaging in the form of 18F-fluorodeoxyglucose (FDG) PET in patients with polymyalgia rheumatica has had a significant impact on the diagnostic work-up of this disorder. This article summarizes the role of FDG-PET imaging in polymyalgia rheumatica with a specific focus on findings, sensitivity and specificity, diagnosis and follow-up, assessment of concurrent large vessel vasculitis, and differential diagnosis.

FDG-PET/CT has potential in inflammatory bowel disease. The literature generally presents good sensitivity and specificity in various settings. At present, the most promising roles are assessment of early treatment response and stricture characterization, whereas general use in the initial diagnostic workup should be reserved for equivocal cases for the time being. However, it is challenging to image the moving and physiologically active bowel with FDG, and available literature is far from ideal. Thus, several issues remain unclarified, and further data are needed to make firm conclusions on the role of FDG and PET/CT in inflammatory bowel disease.

high for routine clinical application and has additional value to conventional tests. Further research is needed to determine the exact place of ^{18}F-FDG PET in the diagnostic work-up of suspected PJI.

Fluorodeoxyglucose-PET/computed tomography combines the high sensitivity of PET with the excellent spatial resolution provided by computed tomography, making it a potentially powerful tool for capturing and quantifying early vascular diseases. Patients with chronic inflammatory states have an increased risk of cardiovascular events; there is also increased vascular fluorodeoxyglucose uptake seen compared with healthy controls. This review examines the use of fluorodeoxyglucose-PET/computed tomography in assessing low-grade vascular inflammation in chronic inflammation and then reviews fluorodeoxyglucose-PET/computed tomography as a tool in monitoring the efficacy of various treatments known to modulate cardiovascular disease.

This review discusses nuclear imaging of inflammation using molecular probes beyond fluoro-d-glucose, is structured by cellular targets, and focuses on those tracers that have been successfully applied clinically.

The role of fluorodeoxyglucose (FDG)-PET/computed tomography (CT) in tuberculosis (TB) continues to expand in disease detection, assessment of the extent of the disease, and treatment response monitoring. This article reviews available data regarding the use of FDG-PET/CT in patients with TB. A new method of quantification for patients with TB is introduced. This method produces robust parameters that represent the total disease burden.

PET CLINICS

SERIES OF RELATED INTEREST

Advances in Clinical Radiology
Available at: Advancesinclinicalradiology.com
MRI Clinics of North America
Available at: MRI.theclinics.com
Neuroimaging Clinics of North America
Available at: Neuroimaging.theclinics.com
Radiologic Clinics of North America
Available at: Radiologic.theclinics.com

THE CLINICS ARE AVAILABLE ONLINE!
Access your subscription at:
www.theclinics.com

PROGRAM OBJECTIVE

The goal of the *PET Clinics* is to keep practicing radiologists and radiology residents up to date with current clinical practice in positron emission tomography by providing timely articles reviewing the state of the art in patient care.

TARGET AUDIENCE

Practicing radiologists, radiology residents, and other health care professionals who provide patient care utilizing radiologic findings.

LEARNING OBJECTIVES

Upon completion of this activity, participants will be able to:
1. Review factors that influence physiological FDG uptake and general FDG distribution that may impact PET/CT imaging in infection and inflammation.
2. Discuss nuclear imaging of inflammation using molecular probes beyond FDG.
3. Recognize the role of ^{18}F-FDG PET for diagnosing infections in prosthetic joints and in the assessment of patients with polymyalgia rheumatica.

ACCREDITATION

The Elsevier Office of Continuing Medical Education (EOCME) is accredited by the Accreditation Council for Continuing Medical Education (ACCME) to provide continuing medical education for physicians.

The EOCME designates this journal-based CME activity for a maximum of 11 *AMA PRA Category 1 Credit*(s)™. Physicians should claim only the credit commensurate with the extent of their participation in the activity.

All other health care professionals requesting continuing education credit for this enduring material will be issued a certificate of participation.

DISCLOSURE OF CONFLICTS OF INTEREST

The EOCME assesses conflict of interest with its instructors, faculty, planners, and other individuals who are in a position to control the content of CME activities. All relevant conflicts of interest that are identified are thoroughly vetted by EOCME for fair balance, scientific objectivity, and patient care recommendations. EOCME is committed to providing its learners with CME activities that promote improvements or quality in healthcare and not a specific proprietary business or a commercial interest.

The planning committee, staff, authors and editors listed below have identified no financial relationships or relationships to products or devices they or their spouse/life partner have with commercial interest related to the content of this CME activity:

Mina Al Najafi, MD; Abass Alavi, MD, MD (Hon), PhD (Hon), DSc (Hon); Sandip Basu, MBBS (Hons), DRM, DNB; Albrecht Betrains, MD; Gregory Bisson, MD, MSCE; Daniel Blockmans, MD, PhD; Jacob Broder Brodersen, MD; Viplav Deogaonkar, MBBS; Amit K. Dey, MD; Lars Christian Gormsen, MD, PhD; Søren Hess, MD; Ashwini Kalshetty, DNB; Marilu Kelly, MSN, RN, CNE, CHCP; Bangkim Chandra Khangembam, MD, FANMB; Malte Kircher, MD; Rakesh Kumar, MD, PhD; Robert M. Kwee, MD, PhD; Thomas C. Kwee, MD, PhD; Constantin Lapa, MD; Aarthi S. Reddy, BS; Asbjørn Mathias Scholtens, MD; Siavash Mehdizadeh Seraj, MD; Domingo E. Ucedam, BS; Mboyo-Di-Tamba Vangu, MD, MMed; John Vassallo, Vignesh Viswanathan

The planning committee, staff, authors and editors listed below have identified financial relationships or relationships to products or devices they or their spouse/life partner have with commercial interest related to the content of this CME activity:

Nehal N. Mehta, MD, MSCE: is a consultant/advisor for and/or received research support from AbbVie Inc., Amgen Inc., Eli Lilly and Company, Celegene Corporation A Bristol-Myers Squibb Company, Janssen Pharmaceuticals, Inc., and Novartis AG

Berit Dalsgaard Nielsen, MD, PhD: participates in a speakers bureau for F. Hoffmann-La Roche Ltd

UNAPPROVED/OFF-LABEL USE DISCLOSURE

The EOCME requires CME faculty to disclose to the participants:
1. When products or procedures being discussed are off-label, unlabelled, experimental, and/or investigational (not US Food and Drug Administration [FDA] approved); and
2. Any limitations on the information presented, such as data that are preliminary or that represent ongoing research, interim analyses, and/or unsupported opinions. Faculty may discuss information about pharmaceutical agents that is outside of FDA-approved labelling. This information is intended solely for CME and is not intended to promote off-label use of these medications. If you have any questions, contact the medical affairs department of the manufacturer for the most recent prescribing information.

TO ENROLL

To enroll in the *PET Clinics* Continuing Medical Education program, call customer service at 1-800-654-2452 or sign up online at http://www.theclinics.com/home/cme. The CME program is available to subscribers for an additional annual fee of USD 235.00.

METHOD OF PARTICIPATION

In order to claim credit, participants must complete the following:

1. Complete enrolment as indicated above
2. Read the activity
3. Complete the CME Test and Evaluation. Participants must achieve a score of 70% on the test. All CME Tests and Evaluations must be completed online

CME INQUIRIES/SPECIAL NEEDS

For all CME inquiries or special needs, please contact elsevierCME@elsevier.com

Preface

Challenging but Clinically Useful: Fluorodeoxyglucose PET/Computed Tomography in Inflammatory and Infectious Diseases

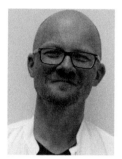
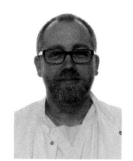

Lars Christian Gormsen, MD, PhD   Søren Hess, MD

Editors

Contemporary fluorodeoxyglucose (FDG) PET/computed tomography (CT) is a valued and integrated part of staging and treatment monitoring of malignant diseases, a development permitted by decades-long massive investment in PET/CT systems by tertiary medical centers worldwide. It was recognized early in the history of PET/CT that as a glucose analogue, FDG was taken up by inflammatory cells as well as by malignant tissue, but initially this nonspecific property of the tracer was considered a nuisance since it caused false positive findings in the oncologic population.[1] Despite early positive reports of FDG-PET imaging used to diagnose bacterial abscesses,[2] promising autoradiography studies demonstrating FDG uptake in neutrophile leukocytes, and evidence of increased glucose transporter activity during inflammation,[3,4] FDG was not widely explored clinically: the nuclear medicine armamentarium already included several much more widely available and allegedly more specific gamma-camera–based infection and inflammation tracers. Nevertheless, in parallel with the increasing demand for oncology FDG-PET/CT scans, excess scanner capacity has gradually allowed for a broader exploration and clinical use of FDG-PET/CT in a range of inflammatory and infectious diseases, such as large vessel vasculitis (LVV), polymyalgia rheumatica

(PMR), sarcoidosis, prosthesis infections, and more heterogeneous entities like fever of unknown origin (FUO).

However, correct acquisition and interpretation of nononcology FDG-PET/CT are associated with several challenges. First, even though a joint European Association of Nuclear Medicine and Molecular Imaging/Society of Nuclear Medicine and Molecular Imaging procedure guideline on FDG-PET/CT for infectious and inflammation is available,[5] optimal scan parameters are still largely unexplored; they are usually extrapolated from the oncologic setting, but the distribution of some infectious or inflammatory diseases may require more focused imaging on specific areas (eg, extremities or cranial arteries). Second, some populations are very heterogeneous, and consequently, scan indications may be just as wide; this is especially evident in FUO with very diverse patient characteristics, definitions, baseline tests, and image interpretation, which renders direct comparison and pooling of data exceedingly difficult. Third, nononcology FDG-PET/CT scans are rarely performed at first presentation of disease; it may in fact be the clinician's last diagnostic resort. As a result, FDG-PET/CT images of inflammatory diseases, for example, reflect widely differing stages of disease, and images consequently may differ

PET Clin 15 (2020) xi–xii
https://doi.org/10.1016/j.cpet.2020.01.002
1556-8598/20/© 2020 Published by Elsevier Inc.

substantially visually. Fourth, since nononcology FDG-PET/CT is typically used as an adjunct imaging technique, patients have often been treated by either corticosteroids or antibiotics prior to referral, which may result in suppression of FDG uptake by inflammatory cells. Fifth, pathologic FDG uptake indicating a specific inflammatory or infectious disease is rarely confirmed by biopsy but rather by clinical outcome.

As a result of these particular challenges, it has been difficult to establish robust threshold values for what constitutes pathologic FDG uptake and also to agree on particular patterns of FDG distribution specific for each inflammatory or infectious disease.

In this issue of *PET Clinics*, we aim to address these problems and present the most up-to-date knowledge of when and how to use FDG-PET/CT in inflammatory and infectious diseases. We have included an initial article detailing correct patient preparation and the caveats associated with concurrent treatment with metformin and corticosteroids (Hess, "Patient Preparation and Patient-Related Challenges in Infectious/Inflammatory Disease"). Optimal use of FDG-PET/CT to diagnose the inflammatory diseases LVV (Nielsen), PMR (Betrains), inflammatory bowel disease (Brodersen), and sarcoidosis (Basu) are discussed in separate articles. Infectious diseases are discussed in articles concerning FUO, bacteremia, and febrile neutropenia (Hess, "Systemic Infections [Fever/Bacteremia of Unknown Origin, Immunocompromised]"), the infected heart (Scholtens), and bone-related infections (Kwee). Finally, 3 articles discuss more experimental approaches to nononcology PET/CT (low-grade inflammation [Reddy], inflammation beyond FDG [Lapa], and quantification in tuberculosis [Deogaonkar]).

As cliché and generic as it may sound, it is imperative that we raise the scientific bar within the overall clinical entity of FDG-PET/CT imaging of infectious and inflammatory diseases. In particular, future efforts should focus on generating valid and robust data from well-designed prospective studies on well-established indications with well-prepared and relevant patient populations.

Lars Christian Gormsen, MD, PhD
Department of Nuclear Medicine &
PET Centre
Aarhus University Hospital
Palle Juul-Jensens Boulevard 165
8200 Aarhus N, Denmark

Søren Hess, MD
Department of Radiology and Nuclear Medicine
Hospital of Southwest Jutland
Finsensgade 35
6700 Esbjerg, Denmark

Department of Regional Health Research
University of Southern Denmark
Odense, Denmark

E-mail addresses:
larsgorm@rm.dk (L.C. Gormsen)
soren.hess@rsyd.dk (S. Hess)

REFERENCES

1. Larson SM. Cancer or inflammation? A Holy Grail for nuclear medicine. J Nucl Med 1994;35(10):1653–5.
2. Tahara T, Ichiya Y, Kuwabara Y, et al. High [18F]-fluorodeoxyglucose uptake in abdominal abscesses: a PET study. J Comput Assist Tomogr 1989;13(5):829–31.
3. Yamada S, Kubota K, Kubota R, et al. High accumulation of fluorine-18-fluorodeoxyglucose in turpentine-induced inflammatory tissue. J Nucl Med 1995;36(7):1301–6.
4. Sugawara Y, Gutowski TD, Fisher SJ, et al. Uptake of positron emission tomography tracers in experimental bacterial infections: a comparative biodistribution study of radiolabeled FDG, thymidine, L-methionine, 67Ga-citrate, and 125I-HSA. Eur J Nucl Med 1999;26(4):333–41.
5. Jamar F, Buscombe J, Chiti A, et al. EANM/SNMMI guideline for 18F-FDG use in inflammation and infection. J Nucl Med 2013;54(4):647–58.

Patient Preparation and Patient-related Challenges with FDG-PET/CT in Infectious and Inflammatory Disease

Søren Hess, MD[a,b,*], Asbjørn Mathias Scholtens, MD[c],
Lars Christian Gormsen, MD, PhD[d]

KEYWORDS

- FDG • PET/CT • Infection • Inflammation • Patient preparation • Physiologic uptake

KEY POINTS

- Physiologic 18F-fluorodeoxyglucose (FDG) uptake and distribution may influence imaging in infection and inflammation and may be counteracted by patient preparation, but recommendations are less established than in malignancy.
- Glucose control is, to a certain degree, probably less important in infection/inflammation than in malignancy.
- Glucocorticoids impairs sensitivity of FDG-PET/CT in large vessel vasculitis and polymyalgia rheumatica and should be discontinued before scan.
- Physiologic bowel activity may be reduced with antiperistaltic drugs and discontinuation of metformin.
- Suppression of myocardial uptake is pivotal in endocarditis and cardiac sarcoidosis and may be achieved by special dietary restrictions and prolonged fasting.

INTRODUCTION

The relative nonspecificity of 18F-fluorodeoxyglucose (FDG) is a multifaceted challenge; accurate differentiation between inflammatory and malignant cells may be difficult because the underlying uptake mechanisms are similar, and physiologic FDG distribution may also influence the diagnostic accuracy. The latter may be counteracted at least to some degree by proper patient preparation, but the potential pitfalls and artifacts may be less pronounced in infectious and inflammatory disease, and there is generally less firm recommendations compared with malignancy. This article outlines some of the challenges with physiologic FDG distribution, and the potential countermeasures to ensure optimal patient preparation before FDG-positron emission tomography/computed tomography (PET/CT) with a focus on infectious and inflammatory diseases, namely the importance of proper glucose control; the potential challenges of ongoing or recent glucocorticoid or metformin treatment; and physiologic FDG distribution in the bowel, urogenital system, and myocardium.

GLUCOSE CONTROL

It is well known that blood glucose levels may influence FDG uptake in malignant cells; for example, as early as 1993, Lindholm and colleagues[1] found

[a] Department of Radiology and Nuclear Medicine, Hospital of Southwest Jutland, Finsensgade 35, Esbjerg 6700, Denmark; [b] Department of Regional Health Research, University of Southern Denmark, Odense, Denmark; [c] Meander Medical Center, Nuclear Medicine, Afd.Nucleaire Geneeskunde, Maatweg 3, Amersfoort 3813 TZ, the Netherlands; [d] Department of Nuclear Medicine & PET Centre, Aarhus University Hospital, Palle Juul-Jensens Boulevard 99, 8200 Aarhus N, Denmark
* Corresponding author. Department of Radiology and Nuclear Medicine, Hospital of Southwest Jutland, Finsensgade 35, 6700 Esbjerg, Denmark.
E-mail address: soeren.hess@rsyd.dk

PET Clin 15 (2020) 125–134
https://doi.org/10.1016/j.cpet.2019.11.001

significantly decreased standardized uptake value (SUV) of tumors as well as overall reduced image quality in 5 patients with head and neck tumors scanned under normal fasting conditions and after oral glucose loading, and Webb and colleagues[2] found maximum SUV values of physiologic liver uptake directly proportional to blood glucose levels. International guidelines prescribe fasting for at least 4 to 6 hours before injection,[3–5] and more specific imaging protocols have been implemented for special indications; for example, imaging of the heart (discussed later). In general, it is suggested to postpone hyperglycemic patients because on-site administration of fast-acting insulin poses other significant challenges; risk of hypoglycemia, interruption of workflow, and decreased image quality caused by increased FDG uptake, especially in skeletal muscle, resulting in a need for repeat scans in as many as 25%[6] (**Fig. 1**). Thus, several schemes have been proposed to counteract hyperglycemia, including personalized insulin calculators,[6] and prescan visits or more strenuous blood glucose sampling,[7] and although these measures successfully reduced the number of postponements, they have not been widely implemented, perhaps because of more challenging logistics.

However, it remains controversial exactly to what extent hyperglycemia affects the diagnostic accuracy of PET imaging in general and whether it also translates into other settings, such as infection and inflammation. For instance, Li and colleagues[8] examined 872 routine PET scans and found potential artifacts in 664 patients (76%), but the cause was postprandial or hyperglycemic in only 21 cases (2,4%) with no impact on final diagnosis, although blood glucose levels were not detailed. Rosica and colleagues[9] found only mild or negligible effects of hyperglycemia of up to 200 mg/dL (11.1 mmol/L) in 325 oncologic patients, with the greatest effect on brain mean SUV (SUVmean), and similar results were found in a recent systematic review and meta-analysis of individual SUV measurements in more than 20,000 patients.[10] Furthermore, data suggest that chronic hyperglycemia has less impact than acute hyperglycemia.[11]

Data on inflammatory cells are scarce and contradictory; early studies on mononuclear cells showed no differential uptake relative to glucose levels at concentrations less than 250 mg/dL, whereas uptake decreased in mesothelioma cells with increasing glucose concentrations. In patients, FDG uptake in malignancies was negatively correlated to glucose levels, whereas uptake in inflammatory lesions was positively correlated to increased glucose levels.[12] In contrast, Zhao and colleagues[13] compared relative FDG uptake in malignant cells, *Staphylococcus aureus* infection, and aseptic turpentine-induced inflammation in a rat model; FDG uptake was 2-fold to 3-fold higher in malignant cells compared with both types of inflammation in euglycemic and euinsulinemic controls, whereas uptake decreased significantly in malignant cells with no effect on inflammatory cells in hypoglycemic insulin-loaded rats, and the opposite results were observed in hyperglycemic rats. However, a more recent consecutive clinical study with 123 patients investigated for inflammatory disease and 320 patients investigated for malignancy compared false-negative rates in diabetic or hyperglycemic patients versus normal patients and found hyperglycemia reduced sensitivity in malignancies with no significant differences in patients with infection or inflammation.[14] However, in most cases, glucose levels were not increased beyond the previously mentioned suggested cutoff of 200 mg/dL.

Thus, it seems glucose levels less than 200 mg/dL (11.1 mmol/L) have limited impact on diagnostic accuracy of infection or inflammation, but further studies are needed to more firmly establish the cutoff levels, especially whether glucose levels greater than 200 mg/dL (11.1 mmol/L) should result in postponement.

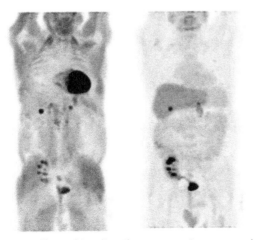

Fig. 1. Effect of insulin. The same patient scanned 2 days apart. (*Left*) The patient had just self-administered fast-acting insulin because of a high plasma glucose level. (*Right*) A few days later under normal blood-glucose conditions. Note again the marked, diffuse FDG uptake in skeletal muscles in the first scan. Liver lesions were present in both scans as well as tracer excretion to a kidney graft. (*From* Basu S, Hess S, Braad P-EN, et al. The Basic Principles of FDG-PET/CT Imaging. PET Clin 2014;355-370; with permission.)

GLUCOCORTICOID THERAPY

By definition, immunosuppressive drugs affect the metabolism of reactive leukocytes and therefore also FDG uptake in inflamed tissue. This wholly anticipated and desired effect unfortunately also significantly affects the efficacy of FDG-PET to aid in diagnosing and monitoring rheumatic diseases once treatment has been initiated. Because referring clinicians tend to institute corticosteroid (CS) treatment of, for example, polymyalgia rheumatica (PMR) or large vessel vasculitis (LVV) based on a clinical diagnosis and only in equivocal cases refer the patient for a confirmatory FDG-PET/CT, several aspects of how CS therapy affects FDG avidity and distribution need to be addressed.

First, it is reasonable to assume that CS therapy does not redistribute the inflammatory cells but rather attenuates their number and metabolic activity. As a consequence, CS therapy most likely only affects the sensitivity and not the specificity of FDG-PET to diagnose inflammatory diseases. This notion is supported by most retrospective studies in which the diagnostic accuracy of FDG-PET/CT to diagnose, for example, LVV has been stratified into steroid-naive and CS-treated patients. Thus, the sensitivity of FDG-PET to diagnose LVV has been reported to decrease from a range of 80% to 95%[15,16] in treatment-naive patients to as low as 33%[17] once high-dose CS therapy has been initiated, whereas specificity remains at ~80% to 90%.[15,17] For PMR, treatment with 8 mg of prednisolone has been shown to reduce the number of sites with FDG avidity indicating bursitis from 9 to 4[18] and therefore also by implication to reduce the sensitivity of FDG-PET/CT.

Prospective and serial studies of FDG uptake in inflamed joints or vessel walls before and after CS treatment are scarce. The authors are only aware of our own study in which a cohort of newly diagnosed giant cell arteritis (GCA) patients with avid vessel wall FDG uptake before CS treatment were rescanned after 3 or 10 days of CS treatment (60 mg of prednisolone). In that study, vessel wall SUVmean was attenuated by ~15% after 3 days of CS treatment, whereas 10 days of treatment reduced SUVmean by 30% to 40%.[19] From a clinical perspective, 3 days of treatment did not affect the visual diagnosis of GCA, whereas 10 days of treatment reduced sensitivity by 60%, results that are in line with the previously mentioned retrospective studies. Thus, a window of opportunity to perform diagnostic FDG-PET seems to exist for the first 3 days of CS treatment, after which the sensitivity decreases rapidly.

Second, it has been shown that CD4+ and CD8+ T cells are particularly susceptible to glucocorticoid-induced apoptosis[20] and that CSs increase macrophage phagocytosis of apoptotic cells, a strongly antiinflammatory process.[21] Rheumatic diseases characterized by strong T-cell responses, such as rheumatoid arthritis (RA), are therefore in theory particularly ill-suited for diagnostic FDG-PET/CT once CS treatment has been initiated. This theory is supported by several studies in which RA-related synovitis and response to short-term treatment with, for example, prednisolone is readily visualized by rapidly decreasing FDG avidity.[22–24]

Third, evidence indicates that the inhibitory effect of CSs on FDG uptake by immune cells may to some extent be dose dependent. In a study by Prieto-Pena and colleagues,[25] patients with treatment-resistant PMR and atypical symptoms were FDG-PET scanned on the suspicion of LVV. Although the patients were treated with an average dose of 12 mg of prednisolone, 60% had vessel wall FDG uptake greater than the liver, indicating coexisting active LVV. Increased large vessel wall FDG uptake has also been observed in a significant proportion of patients with LVV undergoing repeat FDG-PET/CT 3 and 6 months after CS initiation, at which time CS doses had been tapered to within the low dose range.[26] A low prednisolone dose therefore does not seem to significantly inhibit vascular wall immune cell reactivity, and FDG uptake therefore remains avid.

Fourth, CS treatment may also hamper inflammation FDG-PET assessment in a more indirect manner. Although no consensus has been reached as to what amounts to pathologic uptake in, for example, vessel walls or inflamed bursae,[27] most studies have used the liver as a reference organ.[28–30] However, even low-dose CS treatment for as little as 7 to 10 days causes insulin resistance,[31] which results in increasing fasting blood glucose and therefore also in increasing residual FDG activity in the blood pool. As a consequence, the SUV of the highly vascularized liver (the reference organ) increases,[32] further reducing the sensitivity of FDG-PET to diagnose LVV and, in particular, PMR.

In theory, the diagnostic accuracy of FDG-PET to diagnose inflammatory diseases should increase if immunosuppressive therapy is temporarily withheld causing renewed metabolic activity in inflamed target organs. A temporary withdrawal of CS treatment for approximately 2 weeks preceding FDG-PET/CT is therefore recommended by the European Association of Nuclear Medicine (EANM).[33] However, this recommendation is based on theoretic inference because no studies to our knowledge have investigated the impact of CS withdrawal on FDG uptake in inflammatory diseases. That this approach may be feasible is supported mostly by anecdotal evidence and a few case studies. For example, the authors performed 2 FDG-PET scans in a woman with suspected GCA: the first scan was done during high-dose CS treatment and was negative for signs of LVV. The second scan was performed after withholding CS for 14 days, at which time FDG uptake in the aorta was unequivocally increased (**Fig. 2**).

In summary, CS treatment affects the sensitivity but not the specificity of FDG-PET to diagnose LVV and PMR. In addition, it is probable that this effect is dose dependent and any diagnostic FDG-PET/CT should therefore preferably be performed before initiation of CS treatment or at low-dose maintenance (<10 mg of prednisolone).

METFORMIN TREATMENT

Metformin is the endorsed first-line blood glucose level lowering drug prescribed for ~80% of patients with newly diagnosed type 2 diabetes.[34] Because type 2 diabetes is increasing in prevalence and incidence, a significant proportion of patients with suspected inflammatory diseases referred for FDG-PET/CT may also have type 2 diabetes and consequently undergo metformin treatment. Because of metformin's particular mechanism of action, this may pose problems when assessing FDG uptake in the abdominal region and the gastrointestinal tract in particular. Metformin has previously been thought to act primarily by inhibiting hepatic endogenous glucose production[35] but recently this hypothesis has been challenged by some controlled clinical trials as well as clinical FDG-PET/CT experience. Thus, metformin treatment may increase rather than decrease endogenous glucose production in nondiabetic patients[36] and in patients with recent-onset diabetes.[37] In addition, it is a well-known phenomenon that patients treated with metformin have extensive and avid FDG uptake in the gastrointestinal region and in particular in the colonic wall,[38–40] and also that the blood glucose level lowering effect of metformin

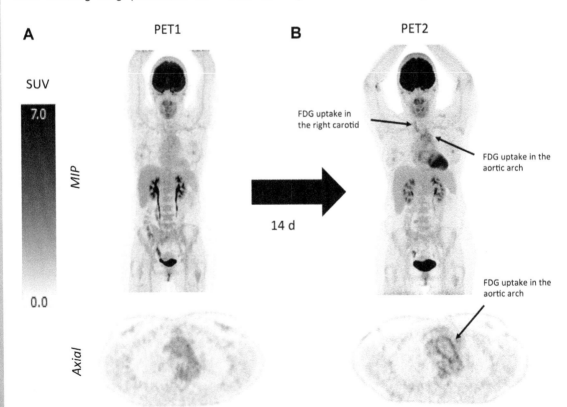

Fig. 2. (*A*) A 51-year-old woman with suspected GCA had been treated with 60 mg of prednisolone for 5 days. C-reactive protein (CRP) level was normal. FDG-PET/CT showed only discrete FDG uptake in the aortic wall (<liver). (*B*) Prednisolone treatment was then withheld for 2 weeks and the patients had repeat FDG-PET/CT. At that time CRP level had increased to 45 mg/L and FDG uptake in the aortic arch and the right carotid was clearly greater than average liver activity. MIP, maximum intensity projection.

correlates well with intestinal FDG uptake.[40] Taken together, these observations indicate that metformin may stimulate enterocyte glucose uptake from the circulation directly, whereby the intestines are in effect turned into an adjunct glucose storage.[41]

From the practical standpoint of an imaging physician, it is important to acknowledge that as little as 7 days of low-dose metformin treatment (500 mg bidaily) increases average colonic FDG activity to greater than liver activity,[42] an effect that is also observed in longer-lasting trials (6 months)[40] and in patients on optimal maintenance dose (1000 mg bidaily).[39] A linear dose-response relationship therefore does not seem to exist. It is also important to realize that metformin treatment seems to increase GI tract wall uptake along an oral-anal gradient, with the most avid uptake in the rectosigmoideal region.[43] Any suspected inflammatory changes in the colon are therefore likely to be obscured by concomitant metformin treatment. This finding has been shown for malignancies, with 2 out of 30 patients treated with metformin having colorectal malignancies obscured by the drug-induced avid colonic FDG uptake.[39] However, withholding metformin treatment for a short period of time can reverse the increased intestinal FDG uptake. In a study of 41 patients with type 2 diabetes, a 3-day halt in metformin treatment decreased FDG uptake in the colon to levels generally observed in comparable nondiabetic subjects.[38] The same was reported by Lee and colleagues,[43] who nicely showed that metformin has to be withheld for 3 days in order for FDG uptake in the rectosigmoideal region to decrease to levels comparable with nontreated subjects. It is important to stress that such a short break in metformin treatment has no adverse long-term consequences for the affected patients' glycemic control and that the short-term consequences are limited to an increase in fasting blood glucose of ~2 to 3 mM.[44] As such, withholding metformin is far less potentially damaging to image interpretation than withholding insulin treatment, which may result in steeply increased fasting blood glucose levels and poor FDG-PET image quality.

In summary, metformin treatment increases intestinal FDG uptake markedly regardless of dosage regimen and should be withheld for 3 days preceding the scheduled PET/CT (**Fig. 3**).

PHYSIOLOGIC ACTIVITY IN THE BOWEL

As mentioned earlier, physiologic activity in the gastrointestinal tract may obscure pathologic findings and hamper interpretation. Underlying mechanisms are incompletely understood but, other than metformin treatment, include involuntary smooth muscle peristalsis, activity in the mucosa and microbial flora, and swallowed or excreted activity. Thus, several potential strategies to attenuate the effects have been suggested or

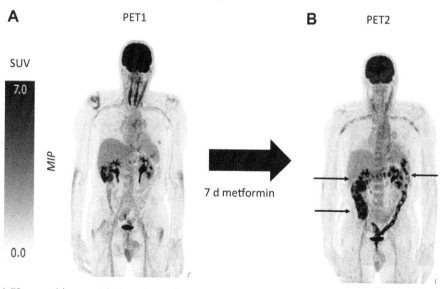

Fig. 3. (*A*) A 72-year-old man with clear signs of arthritis and bursitis. Treated with 60 mg of prednisolone because of suspected LVV. In the course of high-dose CS therapy he developed hyperglycemia and was started on metformin treatment (500 mg bidaily). (*B*) Seven days after initiation of metformin treatment and 3 weeks after the initial PET/CT, he was rescanned because of suspected occult infection. No sign of infection was observed. However, avid FDG uptake was now observed in the colon (*black arrows*). Note also the marked decrease of joint-related FDG uptake and the persistent FDG activity in the lumen of the subclavian and axillary arteries.

attempted, including basic preparatory actions, such as bowel cleansing with isosmotic solutions,[45] varying distension, or filling with water, mannitol, and other contrast agents,[46,47] but most focused on reducing peristalsis. Although mostly evaluated with malignancies in mind, the assessment of possible infection or inflammation, especially in the large intestines, may also be relevant; for example, inflammatory bowel diseases.

Several studies have investigated the antiperistaltic drug N-butylscopolamine, which is already implemented to improve bowel imaging in CT and magnetic resonance imaging colonography.[48] In an in vitro study, Yamamoto and colleagues[49] compared FDG uptake in excised bowel segments from rats and found no statistical differences between those pretreated with N-butylscopolamine and controls. In contrast, Stahl and colleagues[50] evaluated scans in 40 patients with lymphoma, 20 received N-butylscopolamine along with FDG and 20 only received FDG. The groups were compared qualitatively with regard to the extent of activity, with a 4-point grading scale compared with liver uptake, and quantitatively with bowel/liver ratios based on regions of interest. The test group performed significantly better on all accounts; that is, generally lower intensity in fewer regions (1 of 5 vs 2.5 of 5), lower visual scores (1 vs 1.5), and lower bowel/liver ratios (1.5 vs 2.3) compared with the control. Furthermore, bowel uptake only interfered with interpretation in 1 of 20 patients in the test group compared with 6 of 20 in the control group. These results were corroborated by Emmott and colleagues,[48] who found significant overall reduced bowel uptake and increased reader confidentiality in 32 patients pretreated with N-butylscopolamine immediately before FDG injection compared with 32 matched controls. In a recent study, Zhang and colleagues[46] combined the use of mannitol and N-butylscopolamine: 124 patients were randomly assigned to pretreatment with oral water intake, oral mannitol, oral mannitol combined with 10 mg of N-butylscopolamine, or oral mannitol combined with 20 mg of N-butylscopolamine. They found significantly better distension and less FDG uptake with mannitol plus or minus N-butylscopolamine compared with water alone but also significantly more adverse reactions, especially in the latter group.

Because N-butylscopolamine is not commercially available worldwide (eg, United States), alternative agents have also been explored. In an early study, Jadvar and colleagues[51] investigated the effects of atropine and sincalide, which are both known to interact with gastrointestinal motility: 5 healthy men were submitted to 3 different PET scans on 3 different days in random order; FDG was injected after standard fasting at baseline, 5 minutes after sincalide infusion, and 15 minutes after atropine injection. They found no qualitative differences between studies, and concluded that motility may be of minor importance and instead pointed to mucosal activity. Although the number of subjects was limited and no quantitative or semiquantitative assessments were obtained, similar results were encountered by Murphy and colleagues[52] a decade later using a commercial antimotility agent containing atropine: 68 patients referred for routine PET/CT as part of lymphoma work-up were randomized double blinded 1:1 to intervention or water, and bowel uptake was graded using a 4-point visual grading scale. No significant differences were found between the two groups; there was a tendency toward higher uptake in the intervention arm compared with controls.

In conclusion, results are sparse and equivocal at best. N-butylscopolamine seems promising but further studies are needed, especially in the clinical setting of infection and inflammation, to more firmly establish its potential benefit and practical execution.

PHYSIOLOGIC ACTIVITY IN THE UROGENITAL SYSTEM

Similar to bowel activity, urinary tract activity may also hamper assessment of organs or disorder in the vicinity, and various measures to reduce these artifacts have been proposed and tested from the early days of FDG imaging; for example, Leisure and colleagues,[53] who, more than 2 decades ago, proposed a combination of intravenous saline, Foley catheter, furosemide injection, and retrograde filling of the bladder, and in the ensuing years several variations on this theme have been presented. For instance, simple administration of furosemide before scans leads to better assessment of cervical cancer,[54] bladder cancer,[55] and bladder lymphoma[56] compared with standard protocols without diuretic. Others have focused on additional delayed images after forced diuresis (intravenous saline and diuretics) in patients with equivocal abdominopelvic findings: Wang and colleagues[57] found additional significant foci in 18% of patients, Kamel and colleagues[58] found complete elimination of urinary activity in the lower urinary tract in 97% and determined 50% of equivocal lesions adjacent to the urinary tract to be clinically important true-positive findings, and López-Gandul and colleagues[59] achieved physiologic elimination of urine activity in 65% with confirmation of clinical significance of 35% of equivocal prefurosemide images.

However, as with reduction of bowel activity, no studies are available with regard to the (added) value of reduced urine activity in the setting of infection and inflammation. Furthermore, there is still no consensus on the best strategy in the various protocols presented earlier (eg, amount of fluids, doses of diuretics, timing of diuretic injection relative to FDG injection, and scan time).[53–60]

PHYSIOLOGIC ACTIVITY IN THE MYOCARDIUM

Myocardial energy needs are primarily met by the metabolism of free fatty acids (FFAs) and glucose. In the normal resting state approximately 30% of energy is produced from glucose metabolism, but this is highly variable based on the needs of the myocardium and the general metabolic state of the body. Accordingly, the amount of physiologic uptake of FDG in the heart (mainly the left ventricle because of its higher mass and energy expenditure) is highly variable in concordance with the Randle cycle. When imaging (peri)cardiac infection, minimizing the amount of physiologic uptake is crucial to prevent lesions being indistinguishable from the normal background. Because the uptake of glucose and by proxy FDG is governed by the uniporter protein–facilitated glucose transporter (GLUT) member 4, whereas uptake in inflammatory cells is mediated by GLUT1 and GLUT3, it is possible to selectively target this mechanism to reduce the physiologic uptake in the myocardium to levels less than even the normal activity in the blood pool, revealing inflammatory processes in greater detail. By decreasing carbohydrate availability, ensuring levels of serum insulin as low as possible and increasing the availability of FFAs, the myocardial energy consumption may be shifted toward a higher percentage of FFA metabolism. Although a great number of protocols have been described in the literature, there is little to no standardization at present. In the most comprehensive analysis to date, Osborne and colleagues[61] reported that "Collectively, the available literature supports using a high-fat, no-carbohydrate diet for at least two meals with a fast of 4 to 12 hours prior to 18F-FDG PET imaging and suggests that isolated fasting for less than 12 hours and supplementation with food or drink just prior to imaging should be avoided." In patients that cannot undergo dietary protocols, a prolonged fast of more than 18 hours may be effective as an alternate protocol to suppress myocardial glucose metabolism.[61]

The use of intravenous unfractionated heparin as a bolus before FDG administration, which induces pharmacologic lipolysis and thus increases available serum FFA, is a matter of some debate because studies on the subject have shown varying results.[62–65] In the only study to compare the same dietary preparation with and without added heparin, heparin significantly improved myocardial glucose suppression.[64] The latest update by the Japanese Society of Nuclear Cardiology for FDG-PET/CT imaging of sarcoidosis did not include heparin in their recommendations because of incomplete evidence of its efficacy.[66]

SUMMARY

Several factors that influence physiologic FDG uptake and general FDG distribution may affect PET/CT imaging in infection and inflammation. The general impact of hyperglycemia on the diagnostic performance of FDG-PET/CT is probably less in infection/inflammation than in malignancy, at least with blood glucose levels less than 200 mg/dL (11.1 mmol/L), but it remains unknown whether this is also true with higher glucose levels. Patient preparation may reduce physiologic FDG uptake, but recommendations are less established than in malignancy. Local implementation of various patient preparatory measures should reflect the specific patient population and indications; for example, discontinuing glucocorticoids before scan in LVV and polymyalgia rheumatic, reduction of bowel activity by antiperistaltic drugs and discontinuation of metformin, and suppression of myocardial uptake by special dietary restrictions and prolonged fasting in assessment of endocarditis and cardiac sarcoidosis.

DISCLOSURE

Nothing to disclose.

REFERENCES

1. Lindholm P, Minn H, Leskinen-Kallio S, et al. Influence of the blood glucose concentration on FDG uptake in cancer–a PET study. J Nucl Med 1993;34(1): 1–6.
2. Webb RL, Landau E, Klein D, et al. Effects of varying serum glucose levels on 18F-FDG biodistribution. Nucl Med Commun 2015;36(7):717–21.
3. Boellaard R, Delgado-Bolton R, Oyen WJ, et al. FDG PET/CT: EANM procedure guidelines for tumour imaging: version 2.0. Eur J Nucl Med Mol Imaging 2015;42(2):328–54.
4. Jamar F, Buscombe J, Chiti A, et al. EANM/SNMMI guideline for 18F-FDG use in inflammation and infection. J Nucl Med 2013;54(4):647–58.

5. Delbeke D, Coleman RE, Guiberteau MJ, et al. Procedure guideline for tumor imaging with 18F-FDG PET/CT 1.0. J Nucl Med 2006;47(5):885–95.

6. Pattison DA, MacFarlane LL, Callahan J, et al. Personalised insulin calculator enables safe and effective correction of hyperglycaemia prior to FDG PET/CT. EJNMMI Res 2019;9(1):15.

7. Niccoli-Asabella A, Iuele FI, Merenda N, et al. 18F-FDGPET/CT: diabetes and hyperglycaemia. Nucl Med Rev Cent East Eur 2013;16(2):57–61.

8. Li TR, Tian JH, Wang H, Chen ZQ, Zhao CL. Pitfalls in positron emission tomography/computed tomography imaging: causes and their classifications. Chin Med Sci J 2009 Mar;24(1):12–9.

9. Rosica D, Cheng SC, Hudson M, et al. Effects of hyperglycemia on fluorine-18-fluorodeoxyglucose biodistribution in a large oncology clinical practice. Nucl Med Commun 2018;39(5):417–22.

10. Eskian M, Alavi A, Khorasanizadeh M, et al. Effect of blood glucose level on standardized uptake value (SUV) in (18)F- FDG PET-scan: a systematic review and meta-analysis of 20,807 individual SUV measurements. Eur J Nucl Med Mol Imaging 2019;46(1):224–37.

11. Torizuka T, Clavo AC, Wahl RL. Effect of hyperglycemia on in vitro tumor uptake of tritiated FDG, thymidine, L-methionine and L-leucine. J Nucl Med 1997;38(3):382–6.

12. Zhuang HM, Cortes-Blanco A, Pourdehnad M, et al. Do high glucose levels have differential effect on FDG uptake in inflammatory and malignant disorders? Nucl Med Commun 2001;22(10):1123–8.

13. Zhao S, Kuge Y, Tsukamoto E, et al. Effects of insulin and glucose loading on FDG uptake in experimental malignant tumours and inflammatory lesions. Eur J Nucl Med 2001;28(6):730–5.

14. Rabkin Z, Israel O, Keidar Z. Do hyperglycemia and diabetes affect the incidence of false-negative 18F-FDG PET/CT studies in patients evaluated for infection or inflammation and cancer? A Comparative analysis. J Nucl Med 2010;51(7):1015–20.

15. Fuchs M, Briel M, Daikeler T, et al. The impact of 18F-FDG PET on the management of patients with suspected large vessel vasculitis. Eur J Nucl Med Mol Imaging 2012;39(2):344–53.

16. Soussan M, Nicolas P, Schramm C, et al. Management of large-vessel vasculitis with FDG-PET: a systematic literature review and meta-analysis. Medicine 2015;94(14):e622.

17. Hay B, Mariano-Goulart D, Bourdon A, et al. Diagnostic performance of (18)F-FDG PET-CT for large vessel involvement assessment in patients with suspected giant cell arteritis and negative temporal artery biopsy. Ann Nucl Med 2019;33(7):512–20.

18. Sondag M, Guillot X, Verhoeven F, et al. Utility of 18F-fluoro-dexoxyglucose positron emission tomography for the diagnosis of polymyalgia rheumatica: a controlled study. Rheumatology 2016;55(8):1452–7.

19. Nielsen BD, Gormsen LC, Hansen IT, et al. Three days of high-dose glucocorticoid treatment attenuates large-vessel 18F-FDG uptake in large-vessel giant cell arteritis but with a limited impact on diagnostic accuracy. Eur J Nucl Med Mol Imaging 2018;45(7):1119–28.

20. Coutinho AE, Chapman KE. The anti-inflammatory and immunosuppressive effects of glucocorticoids, recent developments and mechanistic insights. Mol Cell Endocrinol 2011;335(1):2–13.

21. Fadok VA, Bratton DL, Konowal A, et al. Macrophages that have ingested apoptotic cells in vitro inhibit proinflammatory cytokine production through autocrine/paracrine mechanisms involving TGF-beta, PGE2, and PAF. J Clin Invest 1998;101(4): 890–8.

22. Roivainen A, Hautaniemi S, Mottonen T, et al. Correlation of 18F-FDG PET/CT assessments with disease activity and markers of inflammation in patients with early rheumatoid arthritis following the initiation of combination therapy with triple oral antirheumatic drugs. Eur J Nucl Med Mol Imaging 2013;40(3): 403–10.

23. Vijayant V, Sarma M, Aurangabadkar H, et al. Potential of (18)F-FDG-PET as a valuable adjunct to clinical and response assessment in rheumatoid arthritis and seronegative spondyloarthropathies. World J Radiol 2012;4(12):462–8.

24. Sarma M, Vijayant V, Basu S. (18)F-FDG-PET assessment of early treatment response of articular and extra-articular foci in newly diagnosed rheumatoid arthritis. Hell J Nucl Med 2012;15(1): 70–1.

25. Prieto-Pena D, Martinez-Rodriguez I, Loricera J, et al. Predictors of positive (18)F-FDG PET/CT-scan for large vessel vasculitis in patients with persistent polymyalgia rheumatica. Semin Arthritis Rheum 2019;48(4):720–7.

26. Blockmans D, De Ceuninck L, Vanderschueren S, et al. Repetitive 18-fluorodeoxyglucose positron emission tomography in isolated polymyalgia rheumatica: a prospective study in 35 patients. Rheumatology 2007;46(4):672–7.

27. Stellingwerff MD, Brouwer E, Lensen KJ, et al. Different scoring methods of FDG PET/CT in giant cell arteritis: need for standardization. Medicine 2015;94(37):e1542.

28. Hautzel H, Sander O, Heinzel A, et al. Assessment of large-vessel involvement in giant cell arteritis with 18F-FDG PET: introducing an ROC-analysis-based cutoff ratio. J Nucl Med 2008;49(7):1107–13.

29. Meller J, Strutz F, Siefker U, et al. Early diagnosis and follow-up of aortitis with [(18)F]FDG PET and MRI. Eur J Nucl Med Mol Imaging 2003;30(5): 730–6.

30. Lehmann P, Buchtala S, Achajew N, et al. 18F-FDG PET as a diagnostic procedure in large vessel

vasculitis-a controlled, blinded re-examination of routine PET scans. Clin Rheumatol 2011;30(1): 37–42.

31. Petersons CJ, Mangelsdorf BL, Jenkins AB, et al. Effects of low-dose prednisolone on hepatic and peripheral insulin sensitivity, insulin secretion, and abdominal adiposity in patients with inflammatory rheumatologic disease. Diabetes care 2013;36(9): 2822–9.

32. Furuya S, Manabe O, Ohira H, et al. Which is the proper reference tissue for measuring the change in FDG PET metabolic volume of cardiac sarcoidosis before and after steroid therapy? EJNMMI Res 2018; 8(1):94.

33. Slart R. FDG-PET/CT(A) imaging in large vessel vasculitis and polymyalgia rheumatica: joint procedural recommendation of the EANM, SNMMI, and the PET Interest Group (PIG), and endorsed by the ASNC. Eur J Nucl Med Mol Imaging 2018;45(7):1250–69.

34. Matthews DR, Inzucchi SE. ADA/EASD position statement of the treatment of type 2 diabetes: reply to Rodbard HW and Jellinger PS [letter], Scheen AJ [letter] and Ceriello A, Gallo M, Gentile S et al [letter]. Diabetologia 2012;55(10):2856–7.

35. Hundal RS, Krssak M, Dufour S, et al. Mechanism by which metformin reduces glucose production in type 2 diabetes. Diabetes 2000;49(12):2063–9.

36. Christensen MM, Hojlund K, Hother-Nielsen O, et al. Endogenous glucose production increases in response to metformin treatment in the glycogen-depleted state in humans: a randomised trial. Diabetologia 2015;58(11):2494–502.

37. Gormsen LC, Sondergaard E, Christensen NL, et al. Metformin increases endogenous glucose production in non-diabetic individuals and individuals with recent-onset type 2 diabetes. Diabetologia 2019; 62(7):1251–6.

38. Ozulker T, Ozulker F, Mert M, et al. Clearance of the high intestinal (18)F-FDG uptake associated with metformin after stopping the drug. Eur J Nucl Med Mol Imaging 2010;37(5):1011–7.

39. Oh JR, Song HC, Chong A, et al. Impact of medication discontinuation on increased intestinal FDG accumulation in diabetic patients treated with metformin. AJR Am J Roentgenol 2010;195(6):1404–10.

40. Koffert JP, Mikkola K, Virtanen KA, et al. Metformin treatment significantly enhances intestinal glucose uptake in patients with type 2 diabetes: results from a randomized clinical trial. Diabetes Res Clin Pract 2017;131:208–16.

41. Rena G, Hardie DG, Pearson ER. The mechanisms of action of metformin. Diabetologia 2017;60(9): 1577–85.

42. Bahler L, Holleman F, Chan MW, et al. 18F-FDG uptake in the colon is modulated by metformin but not associated with core body temperature and energy expenditure. PLoS One 2017;12(5):e0176242.

43. Lee SH, Jin S, Lee HS, et al. Metformin discontinuation less than 72 h is suboptimal for F-18 FDG PET/CT interpretation of the bowel. Ann Nucl Med 2016; 30(9):629–36.

44. Effect of intensive blood-glucose control with metformin on complications in overweight patients with type 2 diabetes (UKPDS 34). UK Prospective Diabetes Study (UKPDS) Group. Lancet 1998; 352(9131):854–65.

45. Miraldi F, Vesselle H, Faulhaber PF, et al. Elimination of artifactual accumulation of FDG in PET imaging of colorectal cancer. Clin Nucl Med 1998;23(1):3–7.

46. Zhang L, Liang ML, Zhang YK, et al. The effects of hypotonic and isotonic negative contrast agent on gastrointestinal distention and physiological intake of 18F-FDG. Nucl Med Commun 2015;36(2):180–6.

47. Sun XG, Huang G, Liu JJ, et al. Comparison of the effect of positive and negative oral contrast agents on (18)F-FDG PET/CT scan. Hell J Nucl Med 2009; 12(2):115–8.

48. Emmott J, Sanghera B, Chambers J, et al. The effects of N-butylscopolamine on bowel uptake: an 18F-FDG PET study. Nucl Med Commun 2008; 29(1):11–6.

49. Yamamoto F, Nakada K, Zhao S, et al. Gastrointestinal uptake of FDG after N-butylscopolamine or omeprazole treatment in the rat. Ann Nucl Med 2004;18(7):637–40.

50. Stahl A, Weber WA, Avril N, et al. Effect of N-butyl-scopolamine on intestinal uptake of fluorine-18-fluorodeoxyglucose in PET imaging of the abdomen. Nuklearmedizin 2000;39(8):241–5.

51. Jadvar H, Schambye RB, Segall GM. Effect of atropine and sincalide on the intestinal uptake of F-18 fluorodeoxyglucose. Clin Nucl Med 1999;24(12): 965–7.

52. Murphy R, Doerger KM, Nathan MA, et al. Pretreatment with diphenoxylate hydrochloride/atropine sulfate (Lomotil) does not decrease physiologic bowel FDG activity on PET/CT scans of the abdomen and pelvis. Mol Imaging Biol 2009; 11(2):114–7.

53. Leisure GP, Vesselle HJ, Faulhaber PF, et al. Technical improvements in fluorine-18-FDG PET imaging of the abdomen and pelvis. J Nucl Med Technol 1997;25(2):115–9.

54. d'Amico A, Gorczewska I, Gorczewski K, et al. Effect of furosemide administration before F-18 fluorodeoxyglucose positron emission tomography/computed tomography on urine radioactivity and detection of uterine cervical cancer. Nucl Med Rev Cent East Eur 2014;17(2):83–6.

55. Nijjar S, Patterson J, Ducharme J, et al. The effect of furosemide dose timing on bladder activity in oncology imaging with 18F-fluorodeoxyglucose PET/CT. Nucl Med Commun 2010;31(2): 167–72.

56. Mantzarides M, Papathanassiou D, Bonardel G, et al. High-grade lymphoma of the bladder visualized on PET. Clin Nucl Med 2005;30(7):478–80.

57. Wang HC, Wang ZM, Wang YB, et al. (18)F-FDG PET/CT delayed images with forced diuresis for revaluating abdominopelvic malignancies. Abdom Radiol (NY) 2017;42(5):1415–23.

58. Kamel EM, Jichlinski P, Prior JO, et al. Forced diuresis improves the diagnostic accuracy of 18F-FDG PET in abdominopelvic malignancies. J Nucl Med 2006;47(11):1803–7.

59. Lopez-Gandul S, Perez-Moure G, Garcia-Garzon JR, et al. Intravenous furosemide injection during 18F-FDG PET acquisition. J Nucl Med Technol 2006;34(4):228–31.

60. Tsai SC, Ou YC, Cheng CL, et al. Reduction of bladder activity on FDG PET/CT scan in patients with urinary bladder carcinoma. A prospective study with a patient-friendly protocol. Nuklearmedizin 2015;54(1):36–42.

61. Osborne MT, Hulten EA, Murthy VL, et al. Patient preparation for cardiac fluorine-18 fluorodeoxyglucose positron emission tomography imaging of inflammation. J Nucl Cardiol 2017;24(1):86–99.

62. Morooka M, Moroi M, Uno K, et al. Long fasting is effective in inhibiting physiological myocardial 18F-FDG uptake and for evaluating active lesions of cardiac sarcoidosis. EJNMMI Res 2014;4(1):1.

63. Manabe O, Yoshinaga K, Ohira H, et al. The effects of 18-h fasting with low-carbohydrate diet preparation on suppressed physiological myocardial (18)F-fluorodeoxyglucose (FDG) uptake and possible minimal effects of unfractionated heparin use in patients with suspected cardiac involvement sarcoidosis. J Nucl Cardiol 2016;23(2):244–52.

64. Scholtens AM, Verberne HJ, Budde RP, et al. Additional heparin preadministration improves cardiac glucose metabolism suppression over low-carbohydrate diet alone in (1)(8)F-FDG PET imaging. J Nucl Med 2016;57(4):568–73.

65. Larson SR, Pieper JA, Hulten EA, et al. Characterization of a highly effective preparation for suppression of myocardial glucose utilization. J Nucl Cardiol 2019. https://doi.org/10.1007/s12350-019-01786-w.

66. Kumita S, Yoshinaga K, Miyagawa M, et al. Recommendations for (18)F-fluorodeoxyglucose positron emission tomography imaging for diagnosis of cardiac sarcoidosis-2018 update: Japanese Society of Nuclear Cardiology recommendations. J Nucl Cardiol 2019;26(4):1414–33.

18F-Fluorodeoxyglucose PET/Computed Tomography in the Diagnosis and Monitoring of Giant Cell Arteritis

Berit Dalsgaard Nielsen, MD, PhD[a,b,c,d,*], Lars Christian Gormsen, MD, PhD[b,c]

KEYWORDS

• Giant cell arteritis • Large vessel vasculitis • 18F-FDG-PET/CT • Diagnostic imaging

KEY POINTS

• Large vessel vasculitis (LVV) can be accurately diagnosed by 18F-fluorodeoxyglucose (FDG)/PET computed tomography (CT); however, sensitivity decreases rapidly after institution of steroid treatment.
• FDG-PET/CT in patients suspected of giant cell arteritis should be performed as a whole-body scan. Assessment should include aorta, aortic main , and extracranial cephalic arteries.
• A homogeneous segmental FDG uptake higher than liver uptake in aorta, its main branches, and/or surrounding tissue in cranial arteries is consistent with LVV.
• Arterial FDG uptake with lower uptake intensity or a different distribution pattern should raise suspicion of alternative diagnoses other than primary LVV.
• Sustained arterial FDG uptake is seen in many patients with LVV despite clinical remission. Accordingly, FDG-PET/CT is not yet suitable for monitoring disease activity.

INTRODUCTION

Giant cell arteritis (GCA) is an autoimmune disease, causing systemic inflammation of large and medium-sized vessels in the elderly (age>50 years) Attempting to determine the diagnosis of GCA can be a challenge. There is no individual pathognomonic symptom or finding by which the diagnosis can be established. Previously, a temporal artery biopsy (TAB) was considered the only confirmatory diagnostic test in GCA and, by definition, was considered specific for GCA. However, diagnostic criteria for a positive TAB are not well defined.[1,2] Moreover, a TAB only has a moderate sensitivity and false-negative biopsy rates ranging from 15% to 66% have been reported.[3,4] Immediate treatment is required in GCA and, because histopathology procedures are time consuming, TABs only rarely alter disease management and are considered by some

---

[a] Department of Rheumatology, Aarhus University Hospital, Palle Juul-Jensens Boulevard 59, Entrance E, Aarhus, Aarhus N 8200, Denmark; [b] Department of Clinical Medicine, Aarhus University, Aarhus, Denmark; [c] Department of Nuclear Medicine and PET Centre, Aarhus University Hospital, Palle Juul-Jensens Boulevard 165, Entrance J, Aarhus 8200, Denmark; [d] Diagnostic Centre, Silkeborg Regional Hospital, Falkevej 1A, 8600 Silkeborg, Denmark
* Corresponding author. Diagnostic Centre, Silkeborg Regional Hospital, Falkevej 1A, 8600 Silkeborg, Denmark.
E-mail address: bernil@rm.dk

PET Clin 15 (2020) 135–145
https://doi.org/10.1016/j.cpet.2019.11.007
1556-8598/20/© 2019 Elsevier Inc. All rights reserved.

clinicians to be unnecessary in patients highly suspicious for GCA.[5–7]

Over the past decades, imaging has become increasingly available in clinical practice and has therefore been extensively studied for GCA diagnosis. Several imaging modalities are now available for confirmation of GCA vessel inflammation.

Recently, European League Against Rheumatism (EULAR) recommendations for the use of imaging in large vessel vasculitis (LVV) in clinical practice recommended that a clinical diagnosis of GCA should be supplemented by an early diagnostic imaging test.[8] The importance of diagnostic imaging in the diagnostic work-up is emphasized by the Diagnosis and Classification in Vasculitis Study validation cohort study, which showed that diagnostic imaging was more likely performed in patients not fulfilling the 1990 classification criteria for GCA (**Box 1**). Modified diagnostic criteria allowing imaging confirmation of GCA diagnosis as a substitute for TAB have also been applied in randomized controlled trials.[9,10]

This article reviews the role of 18F-fluorodeoxyglucose (FDG) PET/computed tomography (CT) in LVV diagnosis and disease monitoring, mainly focusing on GCA. In particular, the diagnostic accuracy, diagnostic criteria, and the potential pitfalls in the interpretation of large vessel FDG uptake are discussed.

GIANT CELL ARTERITIS

Although GCA is a systemic vasculitis, it has become common to consider GCA as either a primarily cranial subtype (c-GCA), affecting the extracranial cephalic arteries, or primarily a large vessel subtype (LV-GCA), affecting the aorta and/or its main branches.[8,11–14] The 2 disease subsets share the symptoms of systemic inflammation, such as fatigue, weight loss, fever, and/or night sweats. Patients with LV-GCA may also present focal symptoms such as limb claudication, large vessel bruits, or pulselessness, but systemic symptoms may be the only manifestation of LV-GCA. In contrast, patients with c-GCA often present cephalic symptoms such as headache, scalp tenderness, visual disturbances, or jaw claudication. GCA can occur isolated or in combination with polymyalgia rheumatica (PMR).

Blood vessel inflammation potentially compromises blood flow, causing ischemic complications such as vision loss, stroke, and scalp or tongue necrosis. However, the risk of ischemic incidents can be markedly reduced by early initiation of glucocorticoid treatment, which is why GCA is considered an acute condition requiring early diagnosis and treatment. Initial glucocorticoid

---

Box 1
Classification criteria for giant cell arteritis

1990 American College of Radiology (ACR) classification criteria for GCA

Categorize patients with vasculitis as having GCA when meeting 3 of the following 5 criteria:

Age more than 50 years

New onset of localized headache

Temporal artery tenderness or decreased temporal artery pulse

Erythrocyte sedimentation rate (ESR) greater than or equal to 50 mm/h

Positive TAB

Proposed revised classification criteria for GCA

Categorize patients with vasculitis as having GCA when at least 1 item in each of the 4 domains is met:

Age 50 years or older

History of ESR greater than or equal to 50 mm/h

At least 1 of the following:

1. Unequivocal cranial symptoms of GCA (new-onset localized headache, scalp or temporal artery tenderness, ischemia-related vision loss, or otherwise unexplained mouth or jaw pain on mastication)

2. Unequivocal symptoms of PMR (shoulder and/or hip girdle pain associated with inflammatory stiffness)

At least 1 of the following:

1. Temporal artery biopsy revealing features of GCA

2. Evidence of LVV by angiography or cross-sectional imaging study such as magnetic resonance angiography, computed tomography angiography, or PET/CT

Data from Hunder GG, Bloch DA, Michel BA, et al. The American College of Rheumatology 1990 criteria for the classification of giant cell arteritis. Arthritis Rheum. 1990 Aug;33(8):1122-8; and Unizony SH, Dasgupta B, Fisheleva E, et al. Design of the tocilizumab in giant cell arteritis trial. *Int J Rheumatol.* 2013. https://doi.org/10.1155/2013/912562.

---

dose is high and treatment duration often exceeds several years. As a consequence, glucocorticoid-related adverse events are frequent in patients with GCA.[15]

Recently, tocilizumab (TCZ), an interleukin (IL)-6 inhibitor, was approved for the treatment of GCA in combination with a more rapidly tapered glucocorticoid regimen. Several clinical trials of other potentially effective targeted synthetic and biologic disease-modifying antirheumatic drugs in GCA are ongoing.[16]

The high risk of potentially serious glucocorticoid-related adverse events and the cost of new glucocorticoid-sparing drugs, emphasize the need for accurate diagnostic tools. The risk of ischemic GCA complications requiring early treatment stresses the importance of readily available diagnostic modalities.

DIAGNOSTIC ACCURACY OF 18F-FLUORODEOXYGLUCOSE PET/ COMPUTED TOMOGRAPHY IN DIAGNOSING LARGE VESSEL GIANT CELL ARTERITIS

A significant number of studies have evaluated the diagnostic accuracy of FDG-PET/CT in diagnosing GCA, mainly focusing on the identification of inflammation in the aorta and its main branches (ie, the LV-GCA subtype). However, several methodological challenges have hampered the interpretation, generalizability, and clinical implementation of these study results.

First, prospective cohort studies of patients suspected to have GCA with double-blinded evaluation of reference diagnosis and FDG-PET/CT are highly lacking. Most previous diagnostic accuracy studies were retrospective[17–22] or case-control studies[23–27] carrying a high risk of confounding or selection bias. However, in a prospective cohort study of patients suspected to have GCA, a sensitivity of 92% and 71% and a specificity of 85% and 91% was recently reported using TAB or clinical diagnosis as a reference, respectively.[28] A sensitivity of 67% and a specificity of 100% has been reported in another prospective study of patients with suspected GCA using clinical judgment, TAB, or American College of Radiology (ACR) criteria as reference.[29]

Second, several different measurement methodologies have been applied assessing the PET images[17,19,21,22,24,25,27,29–35] (**Box 2**), which has prevented implementation of a standardized approach to image acquisition in clinical practice. Until recently, no consensus recommendation or widely accepted interpretation or diagnostic cutoff for the vessel FDG uptake in GCA diagnosis has been agreed on.

Third, an optimal reference test or criteria for LV-GCA does not exist. Clinical diagnosis, TAB, or fulfillment of 1990 ACR criteria for GCA has therefore been used as reference in diagnostic accuracy studies. However, the 1990 ACR classification criteria for GCA mainly focus on the cranial manifestations of the disease (see **Box 1**), and it is well known that patients with LV-GCA are less

---

Box 2
Assessment methodology applied in 18F-fluorodeoxyglucose PET/computed tomography studies evaluating large vessel inflammation

Visual

- Dichotomous: positive or negative[29–31]
- Grading of FDG uptake intensity: no, low, moderate, high[31]
- Grading of arterial FDG uptake relative to liver FDG uptake with different cutoffs[21,22,27,32,33]

Semiquantitative measures (SUV)

- SUV_{mean}
- Mean of $SUV_{max}(ROI)$[34]
- SUV_{max}[22,25,35]

Target/background ratio

- Target is one of the SUV outputs for the artery segment of interest and background is an SUV (mean or maximum) measure in the:
- Liver[24]
- Lungs
- Arterial blood pool[35]
- Venous blood pool[17,19]

$SUV = FDG_{ROI}[Bq/g]/(FDG_{injected\ dose}[Bq]/body\ weight\ [g])$, in a region of interest (ROI) containing the vessel wall and its lumen. *Abbreviations:* Bq, becquerel; ROI, region of interest; SUV, standardized uptake value.

---

likely to have cranial symptoms,[12,36–41] are typically TAB negative,[36,39] and less often fulfill the 1990 ACR criteria for GCA.[12,37,39,40] Consequently, these reference standards may not include all patients with LV-GCA. Using the clinical diagnosis as a reference has for other studies induced a risk of dependency between index test and reference diagnosis.[25,26,32,33]

Despite the great variety in interpretation of PET images and lack of an ideal LV-GCA reference standard, FDG-PET/CT has consistently shown high diagnostic accuracy in GCA. Meta-analyses have revealed sensitivities of 80% to 90% and specificities of 89% to 98%[42–44] using ACR criteria as a reference standard. However, it is noteworthy that the sensitivity of FDG-PET/CT is greatly affected by immunosuppression. Serial FDG-PET/CT performed before and after either 3 or 10 days of high-dose steroids has shown decreasing FDG uptake after institution of treatment. However, diagnostic sensitivity was maintained within 3 days, whereas only about one-third of the patients rescanned after 10 days were still positive. Other studies evaluating diagnostic properties of FDG-PET/CT in mixed populations of treated and untreated patients have also reported that sensitivity is lower in treated patients compared with untreated ones.[17,23,26,27,32,45]

In patients with GCA, the initiation of treatment may not be delayed by diagnostic procedures, because of the risk of ischemic complications. An efficient collaboration between nuclear medicine physicians and rheumatologists is therefore essential in order to prioritize timely diagnostic scans.

DIAGNOSTIC ACCURACY OF 18F-FLUORODEOXYGLUCOSE PET/ COMPUTED TOMOGRAPHY IN DIAGNOSING CRANIAL GIANT CELL ARTERITIS

Although EULAR recommendations do not suggest FDG-PET/CT for the diagnosis of c-GCA, recent publications have revealed that modern PET systems readily detect cranial artery inflammation in patients with GCA.

When PET was first recognized as a potential tool for the diagnosis of GCA, it was reported that FDG-PET/CT could not detect inflammation in the cranial arteries[30] because of (1) poor image resolution, (2) the vessels' juxtaposition to the skin-air interface, and (3) spill-in from physiologic cerebral brain FDG uptake. However, the authors recently performed a case-control study in which a sensitivity of 82% and a specificity of 100% was found for the diagnosis of c-GCA by conventional FDG-PET/CT. In the cranial arteries, FDG uptake in the temporal, maxillary, or vertebral arteries above the surrounding tissue was considered positive and thus to indicate c-GCA. High interrater agreement was obtained in spite of assessment performed by nuclear medicine physicians after only a brief training session lasting 30 minutes. Also, cranial PET was not inferior to TAB.[46] The high sensitivity of cranial artery assessment has subsequently been confirmed in a prospective study of patients suspected to have GCA. FDG uptake in cephalic arteries was reported in 75% of patients with TAB-positive GCA. FDG uptake in cephalic arteries was only reported in 2% of the control patients, indicating a high specificity also in controls suspected to have GCA.[28] A few case reports have also described FDG uptake in cephalic arteries in patients with GCA.[47–50] These findings indicate that the combination of PET with CT and the improved resolution of newer PET systems allow c-GCA diagnosis by PET and suggest that, in patients suspected of having GCA, FDG-PET/CT should include the head and neck.

DEFINITIONS OF VASCULAR 18F-FLUORODEOXYGLUCOSE PET/ COMPUTED TOMOGRAPHY LESIONS AND RELIABILITY

A homogeneous segmental high-intensity FDG uptake in large vessels is considered consistent with LVV (**Fig. 1**). As described earlier, the acquisition of PET images in previous studies has been inconsistent, as has the diagnostic cutoff to consider FDG uptake indicative of vasculitis. Therefore, procedural guidelines for image assessment and diagnostic criteria regarding FDG intensity and distribution have been in high demand. Recently, a joint procedural recommendation was published on the use of FDG-PET/CT in LVV and PMR developed by the European Association of Nuclear Medicine, the Society of Nuclear Medicine and Molecular Imaging, and the PET Interest Group, and it was endorsed by the American Society of Nuclear Cardiology.[51] The recommendations encompass patient preparation, FDG-PET/CT image acquisition as well as interpretation, and it is hoped that it will ensure that uniform procedures are used in daily clinical practice and in clinical trials. This process will facilitate optimal diagnostic accuracy and comparative study designs.

Based on available literature and expert consensus, recommendations advocate that, for the clinical diagnosis, FDG uptake in aorta and its main branches is graded according to liver FDG uptake (grade 0, no vascular uptake; grade 1, vascular uptake <liver uptake; grade 2, vascular uptake equal to liver uptake; grade 3, vascular uptake greater than liver uptake). Grade 3 is considered consistent with vasculitis, whereas grade 2 be indicate vasculitis. A visual grading of vessel FDG uptake relative to liver uptake is quick and feasible for clinical implementation and also has shown high reproducibility and high interrater agreement.[17,18,21,26] The grade 3 conservative cutoff has shown high diagnostic accuracy in studies comparing different interpretations and cutoffs (**Fig. 1**).[17,18]

Although LV-GCA may involve aorta, its main branches, and cephalic medium-sized extracranial arteries, not all branches have to be involved.[51] A typical topographic GCA pattern is the involvement of aorta and/or supra-aortic branches with or without the involvement of infra-aortic arteries.[21,34,37,41,52–55] On FDG-PET/CT, the best discrimination between patients with GCA and controls is obtained in the supra-aortic region, whereas FDG uptake in the aorta and infra-aortic regions is much less specific.[45] Isolated involvement of infra-aortic arteries or the aorta does not

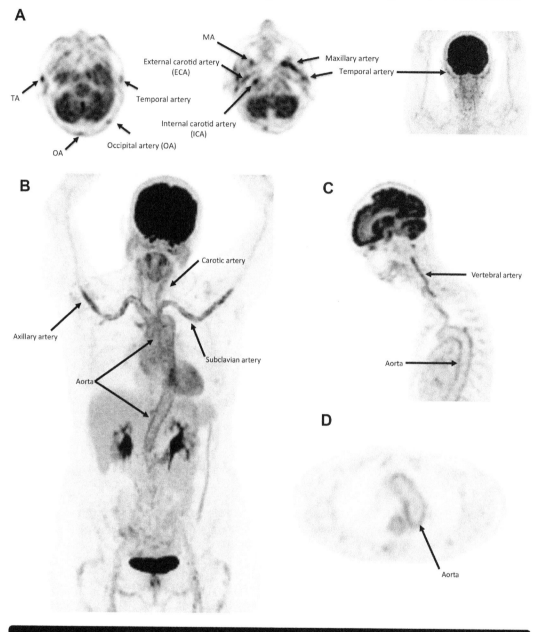

Typical PET features of giant cell arteritis

Pattern	Distribution	Intensity
• Segmental	• Aorta, aortic main branches, extracranial cephalic arteries.	Aorta and aortic large branches:
• Circumferential	• Not all vessels needs to be involved	• Arterial FDG uptake higher than liver uptake
• Homogeneous	• Supra-aortic and cephalic arteries being most specific	Cephalic extracranial arteries (incl. vertebral):
		• FDG uptake higher than surrounding tissue

Fig. 1. Typical FDG-PET/CT features of GCA. Maximal intensity projection images showing (*A*) examples of increased FDG uptake in different cephalic arteries in patients with GCA; (*B*) typical large vessel GCA with a smooth concentric, segmental, and homogeneous arterial FDG uptake higher than liver FDG uptake in the aorta, brachiocephalic trunk, subclavian, and carotid and axillary arteries; (*C*) homogeneous, segmental increased FDG uptake in vertebral arteries and aorta in a patient with GCA and (*D*) in aortic arch of a patient with GCA. MA, maxillary artery; OA, ociipital artery; TA, temporal artery.

exclude GCA,[38] but care must be taken not to mistake severe atherosclerosis for LV-GCA.[21–23] In atherosclerotic vessels, subendothelial smooth muscle proliferation or activated macrophages within plaques may cause low-grade, often patchy or focal FDG uptake.[17,56]

Large vessel inflammation may also be seen in conditions other than primary vasculitis. For example, aortitis is also seen in some patients with rheumatoid arthritis, Cogan syndrome, relapsing polychondritis, ankylosing spondylitis, systemic lupus erythematosus, Buerger disease, Behçet disease, inflammatory bowel disease, sarcoidosis, retroperitoneal fibrosis, immunoglobulin G4 disease, syphilis, and tuberculosis.[57–59] Therefore, differential diagnoses must be considered in patients not presenting with typical GCA symptoms and/or an atypical distribution of vessel involvement (**Fig. 2**).

VALUE OF 18F-FLUORODEOXYGLUCOSE PET/ COMPUTED TOMOGRAPHY COMPARED WITH OTHER IMAGING MODALITIES

FDG-PET/CT has several advantages making it valuable for LVV diagnosis. PET is a cross-sectional imaging technique that usually covers the entire body from skull to thigh and hence potentially visualizes all inflamed vessels large enough to be detected by the PET system. FDG-PET identifies areas of high glucose uptake by measuring the amount of tracer in the nanomolar to picomolar range. The detection of a molecular process makes it possible to identify disease activity that has not yet caused morphologic vessel changes detectable by more conventional imaging techniques. Combining PET with CT allows attenuation correction and high-resolution visualization of anatomic structures. FDG-PET/CT also has the major advantage of evaluating potential differential diagnoses such as malignancy or infection that GCA may imitate.

In contrast, FDG-PET/CT is labor intensive, requires some patient preparation (fasting and peripheral venous catheter), and is based on the use of ionizing radiation. Moreover, FDG-PET/CT may not be readily available in smaller hospitals. Hence, FDG-PET/CT is not an obvious first-line examination to be performed in all patients suspected to have GCA.

Based on an extensive literature review and meta-analysis on imaging in LVV,[60] EULAR recommendations for the use of imaging in LVV in clinical practice suggest vascular ultrasonography (US) as a first-line imaging test for patients suspected of having c-GCA. However, US may also be used for confirmation of large vessel inflammation. The diagnostic accuracy of US for c-GCA is well established, whereas the added value of examining large vessels is less explored.

The diagnostic yield of US using PET as a reference was evaluated in a retrospective study of 50 patients suspected of having LVV of different causes. A sensitivity of 80% and specificity of 70% was found for the overall LVV diagnosis. Analyzing each artery separately, the highest accuracy was obtained in the axillary and subclavian arteries and the lowest in the abdominal aorta, visceral branches, and femoral artery.[61]

A good agreement between US and FDG-PET findings of LVV has been found in smaller GCA cohorts.[21,25,30,62] Although these studies indicate a promising role for US in the diagnosis of LV-GCA, it is noticeable that FDG-PET/CT detects large vessel inflammation in 80% to 90% of patients with GCA,[51] whereas US studies usually report large vessel inflammation in only about 30% to 50%.[37,40,52,63–68]

CT angiography may also be used for confirmation of large vessel inflammation[34,69] and seems to correlate well with FDG-PET–proven LVV.[29,70,71] Conventional CT scans are often performed early in the disease course because of unspecific constitutional symptoms raising suspicion of malignancy. In these patients, conventional CT often identifies vessel wall thickening instead, indicating LVV.[72]

However, for most studies comparing different imaging modalities, the cohorts investigated were often selected based on either clinical or imaging findings of large vessel involvement, hence inducing possible selection bias or circular reasoning.

CAN 18F-FLUORODEOXYGLUCOSE PET/ COMPUTED TOMOGRAPHY BE USED TO MONITOR DISEASE ACTIVITY IN GIANT CELL ARTERITIS?

Recalling the high risk of adverse events from glucocorticoid treatment, avoiding complications and maintaining disease remission with the lowest possible glucocorticoid dose is the target of GCA treatment. According to guidelines, glucocorticoid is subsequently tapered and discontinuation is aimed for after 1 to 2 years of treatment.[73–75] Disease flares during tapering are frequent and the need for several years of glucocorticoid treatment is common.[76–79] The approval of TCZ as a steroid-sparing add-on drug has further strengthened clinicians' obligation to avoid glucocorticoid overtreatment.

Biomarkers of disease activity and prognosis to guide GCA treatment are lacking. Assessment of

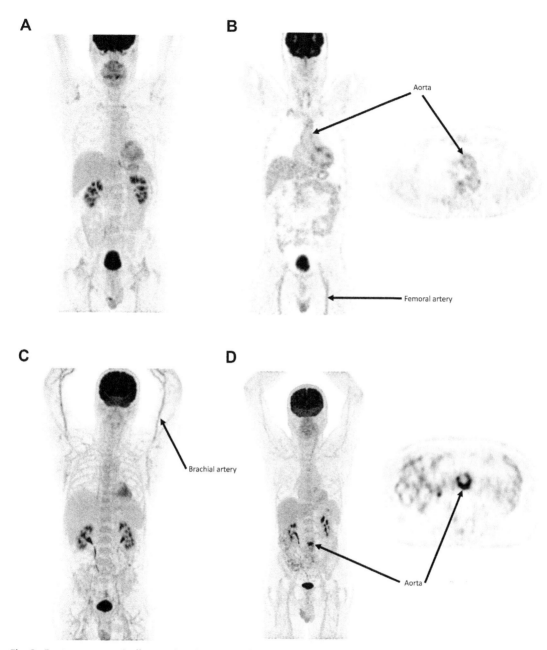

Fig. 2. Features not typically seen in primary LVV. (*A*) Normal FDG-PET/CT without increased vascular FDG uptake. (*B*) Focal, patchy aortic and femoral arterial FDG uptake less than or equal to liver FDG uptake consistent with atherosclerosis. (*C*) Increased FDG uptake greater than liver FDG uptake in peripheral large arm arteries but not in proximal main branches of aorta, in aorta, or in cephalic arteries in a patient with fever and increased levels of inflammatory markers. Symptoms and inflammatory biomarkers spontaneously normalized within a few weeks. (*D*) Focal high-intensity uptake in abdominal aorta and surrounding soft tissue in a patient with retroperitoneal fibrosis.

disease activity is based on the clinician's interpretation of unspecific symptoms and traditional biomarkers of inflammation, making glucocorticoid overtreatment, and consequently glucocorticoid toxicity, unavoidable. For patients in TCZ treatment, traditional acute phase reactants are even less useful.[80] Therefore, there is an unmet need for monitoring biomarkers in GCA.

FDG-PET/CT is a valuable tool to monitor treatment response in various cancers, notably lymphomas, for which it is part of routine clinical evaluation of chemoresponsiveness and prognostication.[81] In

LVV, FDG-PET/CT has also been studied as a potential tool to assess disease activity. Although immunosuppressive treatment decreases FDG uptake,[35,82–84] a significant number of patients with LVV considered in clinical and biochemical remission surprisingly show persistent vascular FDG uptake during follow-up.[31,85–87] Also, on follow-up scans, semiquantitative measures of FDG uptake cannot distinguish clinically active from inactive disease.[35] Similar findings of persistent vessel wall thickening otherwise considered indicative of vasculitis in the diagnostic evaluation of LVV have been reported for other imaging modalities during clinical remission.[86,88,89] In contrast, vascular FDG uptake at baseline has been shown to be associated with a higher risk of subsequent relapse and a higher risk of aortic dilatation,[85,90] and may also be a promising biomarker of treatment response for study purposes.[91] Further studies are needed to clarify the relevance of PET as a supporting tool for clinical decision making during the disease course.

In conclusion, FDG-PET/CT is a valuable tool for the confirmation of LVV. To ensure high diagnostic accuracy, the arterial FDG uptake in aorta, aortic branches, and cephalic arteries must be evaluated and intensity, patterns, and distribution must be critically interpreted by both the assessor and the clinician, who must be aware of potential pitfalls and differential diagnosis. In contrast, FDG-PET/CT is not recommended for the assessment of disease activity. Further studies are awaited to confirm PET as a potential prognostic biomarker.

DISCLOSURE

B.D. Nielsen has received fees for speaking from Roche.

REFERENCES

1. Stacy RC, Rizzo JF, Cestari DM. Subtleties in the histopathology of giant cell arteritis. Semin Ophthalmol 2011;26(4–5):342–8.
2. Banz Y, Stone JH. Why do temporal arteries go wrong? Principles and pearls from a clinician and a pathologist. Rheumatology 2018;57(suppl_2):ii3–10.
3. Ashton-Key MR, Gallagher PJ. False-negative temporal artery biopsy. Am J Surg Pathol 1992;16(6):634.
4. Germanò G, Muratore F, Cimino L, et al. Is colour duplex sonography-guided temporal artery biopsy useful in the diagnosis of giant cell arteritis? A randomized study. Rheumatology (Oxford) 2015;54(3):400–4.
5. Chong EWT, Robertson AJ. Is temporal artery biopsy a worthwhile procedure? ANZ J Surg 2005;75(6):388–91.
6. Quinn EM, Kearney DE, Kelly J, et al. Temporal artery biopsy is not required in all cases of suspected giant cell arteritis. Ann Vasc Surg 2012;26(5):649–54.
7. Bowling K, Rait J, Atkinson J, et al. Temporal artery biopsy in the diagnosis of giant cell arteritis: does the end justify the means? Ann Med Surg 2017;20:1–5.
8. Dejaco C, Ramiro S, Duftner C, et al. EULAR recommendations for the use of imaging in large vessel vasculitis in clinical practice. Ann Rheum Dis 2018;77(5):636–43.
9. Langford CA, Cuthbertson D, Ytterberg SR, et al. A randomized, double-blind trial of abatacept (CTLA-4Ig) for the treatment of giant cell arteritis. Arthritis Rheumatol 2017;69(4):837–45.
10. Unizony SH, Dasgupta B, Fisheleva E, et al. Design of the tocilizumab in giant cell arteritis trial. Int J Rheumatol 2013. https://doi.org/10.1155/2013/912562.
11. Dejaco C, Duftner C, Buttgereit F, et al. The spectrum of giant cell arteritis and polymyalgia rheumatica: revisiting the concept of the disease. Rheumatology (Oxford) 2017;56(4):506–15.
12. Muratore F, Kermani TA, Crowson CS, et al. Large-vessel giant cell arteritis: a cohort study. Rheumatology (Oxford) 2015;54(3):463–70.
13. de Boysson H, Lambert M, Liozon E, et al. Giant-cell arteritis without cranial manifestations. Medicine (Baltimore) 2016;95(26):e3818.
14. Koster MJ, Matteson EL, Warrington KJ. Large-vessel giant cell arteritis: diagnosis, monitoring and management. Rheumatology 2018;57(suppl_2):ii32–42.
15. Proven A, Gabriel SE, Orces C, et al. Glucocorticoid therapy in giant cell arteritis: duration and adverse outcomes. Arthritis Rheum 2003;49(5):703–8.
16. Dejaco C, Brouwer E, Mason JC, et al. Giant cell arteritis and polymyalgia rheumatica: current challenges and opportunities. Nat Rev Rheumatol 2017;13(10):1–15.
17. Stellingwerff MD, Brouwer E, Lensen K-JDF, et al. Different scoring methods of FDG PET/CT in giant cell arteritis: need for standardization. Medicine (Baltimore) 2015;94(37):e1542.
18. Lensen KDF, Comans EFI, Voskuyl AE, et al. Large-vessel vasculitis: interobserver agreement and diagnostic accuracy of 18F-FDG-PET/CT. Biomed Res Int 2015. https://doi.org/10.1155/2015/914692.
19. Besson FL, De Boysson H, Parienti JJ, et al. Towards an optimal semiquantitative approach in giant cell arteritis: an 18F-FDG PET/CT case-control study. Eur J Nucl Med Mol Imaging 2014;41(1):155–66.
20. Yamashita H, Kubota K, Takahashi Y, et al. Whole-body fluorodeoxyglucose positron emission

tomography/computed tomography in patients with active polymyalgia rheumatica: evidence for distinctive bursitis and large-vessel vasculitis. Mod Rheumatol 2012;22(5):705–11.

21. Förster S, Tato F, Weiss M, et al. Patterns of extracranial involvement in newly diagnosed giant cell arteritis assessed by physical examination, colour coded duplex sonography and FDG-PET. Vasa 2011;40(3):219–27.

22. Lehmann P, Buchtala S, Achajew N, et al. 18F-FDG PET as a diagnostic procedure in large vessel vasculitis-a controlled, blinded re-examination of routine PET scans. Clin Rheumatol 2011;30(1):37–42.

23. Prieto-González S, Depetris M, García-Martínez A, et al. Positron emission tomography assessment of large vessel inflammation in patients with newly diagnosed, biopsy-proven giant cell arteritis: a prospective, case–control study. Ann Rheum Dis 2014;73(7):1388–92.

24. Hautzel H, Sander O, Heinzel A, et al. Assessment of large-vessel involvement in giant cell arteritis with 18F-FDG PET: introducing an ROC-analysis-based cutoff ratio. J Nucl Med 2008;49(7):1107–13.

25. Henes JC, Müller M, Krieger J, et al. [18F] FDG-PET/CT as a new and sensitive imaging method for the diagnosis of large vessel vasculitis. Clin Exp Rheumatol 2008;26:S47–52.

26. Walter MA, Melzer RA, Schindler C, et al. The value of [18F]FDG-PET in the diagnosis of large-vessel vasculitis and the assessment of activity and extent of disease. Eur J Nucl Med Mol Imaging 2005;32(6):674–81.

27. Clifford AH, Murphy EM, Burrell SC, et al. Positron emission tomography/computerized tomography in newly diagnosed patients with giant cell arteritis who are taking glucocorticoids. J Rheumatol 2017;44(12):1859–66.

28. Sammel AM, Hsiao E, Schembri G, et al. Diagnostic accuracy of PET/CT scan of the head, neck and chest for giant cell arteritis: the double-blinded giant cell arteritis and PET scan (GAPS) study. Arthritis Rheumatol 2019. https://doi.org/10.1002/art.40864.

29. Lariviere D, Benali K, Coustet B, et al. Positron emission tomography and computed tomography angiography for the diagnosis of giant cell arteritis. Medicine (Baltimore) 2016;95(30):e4146.

30. Brodmann M, Lipp RW, Passath A, et al. The role of 2-18F-fluoro-2-deoxy-D-glucose positron emission tomography in the diagnosis of giant cell arteritis of the temporal arteries. Rheumatology 2004;43(2):241–2.

31. Blockmans D, de Ceuninck L, Vanderschueren S, et al. Repetitive 18F-fluorodeoxyglucose positron emission tomography in giant cell arteritis: a prospective study of 35 patients. Arthritis Rheum 2006;55(1):131–7.

32. Fuchs M, Briel M, Daikeler T, et al. The impact of 18F-FDG PET on the management of patients with suspected large vessel vasculitis. Eur J Nucl Med Mol Imaging 2012;39(2):344–53.

33. Blockmans D, Stroobants S, Maes A, et al. Positron emission tomography in giant cell arteritis and polymyalgia rheumatica: evidence for inflammation of the aortic arch. Am J Med 2000;108(3):246–9.

34. Prieto-González S, Arguis P, García-Martínez A, et al. Large vessel involvement in biopsy-proven giant cell arteritis: prospective study in 40 newly diagnosed patients using CT angiography. Ann Rheum Dis 2012;71(7):1170–6.

35. Martínez-Rodríguez I, Martínez-Amador N, Banzo I, et al. Assessment of aortitis by semiquantitative analysis of 180-min 18F-FDG PET/CT acquisition images. Eur J Nucl Med Mol Imaging 2014;41(12):2319–24.

36. Brack A, Martinez-Taboada V, Stanson A, et al. Disease pattern in cranial and large-vessel giant cell arteritis. Arthritis Rheum 1999;42(2):311–7.

37. Schmidt WA, Seifert A, Gromnica-ihle E, et al. Ultrasound of proximal upper extremity arteries to increase the diagnostic yield in large-vessel giant cell arteritis. Rheumatology 2008;47(1):96–101.

38. Berti A, Campochiaro C, Cavalli G, et al. Giant cell arteritis restricted to the limb arteries: an overlooked clinical entity. Autoimmun Rev 2015;14(4):352–7.

39. de Boysson H, Daumas A, Vautier M, et al. Large-vessel involvement and aortic dilation in giant-cell arteritis. A multicenter study of 549 patients. Autoimmun Rev 2018;17(4):391–8.

40. Czihal M, Zanker S, Rademacher A, et al. Sonographic and clinical pattern of extracranial and cranial giant cell arteritis. Scand J Rheumatol 2012;41(3):231–6.

41. Kermani TA, Diab S, Sreih AG, et al. Arterial lesions in giant cell arteritis: a longitudinal study. Semin Arthritis Rheum 2020;48(4):707–13.

42. Besson FL, Parienti J-J, Bienvenu B, et al. Diagnostic performance of 18F-fluorodeoxyglucose positron emission tomography in giant cell arteritis: a systematic review and meta-analysis. Eur J Nucl Med Mol Imaging 2011;38(9):1764–72.

43. Soussan M, Nicolas P, Schramm C, et al. Management of large-vessel vasculitis with FDG-PET: a systematic literature review and meta- analysis. Medicine (Baltimore) 2015;94(14):e622.

44. Mackie SL, Arat S, Da Silva J, et al. Polymyalgia rheumatica (PMR) special interest group at OMERACT 11: outcomes of importance for patients with PMR. J Rheumatol 2014;41(4):819–23.

45. Imfeld S, Rottenburger C, Schegk E, et al. [18 F] FDG positron emission tomography in patients presenting with suspicion of giant cell arteritis-lessons from a vasculitis clinic. Eur Heart J Cardiovasc Imaging 2018;19(8):933–40.

46. Nielsen BD, Hansen IT, Kramer S, et al. Simple dichotomous assessment of cranial artery inflammation by conventional 18F-FDG PET/CT shows high accuracy for the diagnosis of giant cell arteritis: a case-control study. Eur J Nucl Med Mol Imaging 2019;46(1):184–93.

47. Rehak Z, Szturz P, Kren L, et al. Upsampling from aorta and aortic branches: PET/CT hybrid imaging identified 18F-FDG hypermetabolism in inflamed temporal and occipital arteries. Clin Nucl Med 2014;39(1):e84–6.

48. Sammel AM, Hsiao E, Nguyen K, et al. Maxillary artery 18F-FDG uptake as a new finding on PET/CT scan in a cohort of 41 patients suspected of having giant cell arteritis. Int J Rheum Dis 2018;21(2):560–2.

49. Sammel AM, Hsiao E, Schrieber L, et al. Fluorine-18 fluoro-2-deoxyglucose positron emission tomography uptake in the superficial temporal and vertebral arteries in biopsy positive giant cell arteritis. J Clin Rheumatol 2017;23(8):443.

50. Maffione AM, Rampin L, Grassetto G, et al. 18F-FDG PET/CT of generalized arteritis. Clin Nucl Med 2018;43(1):48–9.

51. Slart RHJA, Writing Group, Reviewer Group, Members of EANM Cardiovascular, Members of EANM Infection & Inflammation, Members of Committees, SNMMI Cardiovascular, Members of Council, PET Interest Group, Members of ASNC, EANM Committee Coordinator. FDG-PET/CT(A) imaging in large vessel vasculitis and polymyalgia rheumatica: joint procedural recommendation of the EANM, SNMMI, and the PET Interest Group (PIG), and endorsed by the ASNC. Eur J Nucl Med Mol Imaging 2018;45(7):1250–69.

52. Aschwanden M, Kesten F, Stern M, et al. Vascular involvement in patients with giant cell arteritis determined by duplex sonography of 2x11 arterial regions. Ann Rheum Dis 2010;69(7):1356–9.

53. Lie JT. Aortic and extracranial large vessel giant cell arteritis: a review of 72 cases with histopathologic documentation. Semin Arthritis Rheum 1995;24(6):422–31.

54. Schmidt WA, Natusch A, Möller DE, et al. Involvement of peripheral arteries in giant cell arteritis: a color Doppler sonography study. Clin Exp Rheumatol 2002;20:309–18.

55. Grayson PC, Maksimowicz-McKinnon K, Clark TM, et al. Distribution of arterial lesions in Takayasu's arteritis and giant cell arteritis. Ann Rheum Dis 2012;71(8):1329–34.

56. Dunphy MPS, Freiman A, Larson SM, et al. Association of vascular 18 F-FDG uptake with vascular calcification. J Nucl Med 2005;46(8):1278–84.

57. Restrepo CS, Ocazionez D, Suri R, et al. Aortitis: imaging spectrum of the infectious and inflammatory conditions of the aorta. Radiographics 2011;31(2):435–51.

58. Cinar I, Wang H, Stone JR. Clinically isolated aortitis: pitfalls, progress, and possibilities. Cardiovasc Pathol 2017;29:23–32.

59. Hartlage GR, Palios J, Barron BJ, et al. Multimodality imaging of aortitis. JACC Cardiovasc Imaging 2014;7(6):605–19.

60. Duftner C, Dejaco C, Sepriano A, et al. Imaging in diagnosis, outcome prediction and monitoring of large vessel vasculitis: a systematic literature review and meta-Analysis informing the EULAR recommendations. RMD Open 2018;4(1). https://doi.org/10.1136/rmdopen-2017-000612.

61. Löffler C, Hoffend J, Benck U, et al. The value of ultrasound in diagnosing extracranial large-vessel vasculitis compared to FDG-PET/CT: a retrospective study. Clin Rheumatol 2017. https://doi.org/10.1007/s10067-017-3669-7.

62. Czihal M, Tatò F, Förster S, et al. Fever of unknown origin as initial manifestation of large vessel giant cell arteritis: diagnosis by colour-coded sonography and 18-FDG-PET. Clin Exp Rheumatol 2010;28(4):549–52.

63. Diamantopoulos AP, Haugeberg G, Hetland H, et al. Diagnostic value of color Doppler ultrasonography of temporal arteries and large vessels in giant cell arteritis: a consecutive case series. Arthritis Care Res 2014;66(1):113–9.

64. Czihal M, Schröttle A, Baustel K, et al. B-mode sonography wall thickness assessment of the temporal and axillary arteries for the diagnosis of giant cell arteritis: a cohort study. Clin Exp Rheumatol 2017;35(1):128–33.

65. Schäfer VS, Juche A, Ramiro S, et al. Ultrasound cut-off values for intima-media thickness of temporal, facial and axillary arteries in giant cell arteritis. Rheumatology 2017;56(9):1479–83.

66. Ghinoi A, Pipitone N, Nicolini A, et al. Large-vessel involvement in recent-onset giant cell arteritis: a case-control colour-Doppler sonography study. Rheumatology 2012;51(4):730–4.

67. Ješe R, Rotar Ž, Tomšič M, et al. The role of colour Doppler ultrasonography of facial and occipital arteries in patients with giant cell arteritis: a prospective study. Eur J Radiol 2017;95:9–12.

68. Monti S, Floris A, Ponte CB, et al. The proposed role of ultrasound in the management of giant cell arteritis in routine clinical practice. Rheumatology (Oxford) 2018;57(1):112–9.

69. Agard C, Barrier JH, Dupas B, et al. Aortic involvement in recent-onset giant cell (temporal) arteritis: a case-control prospective study using helical aortic computed tomodensitometric scan. Arthritis Care Res 2008;59(5):670–6.

70. de Boysson H, Dumont A, Liozon E, et al. Giant-cell arteritis: concordance study between aortic CT angiography and FDG-PET/CT in detection of large-vessel involvement. Eur J Nucl Med Mol

Imaging 2017;1–6. https://doi.org/10.1007/s00259-017-3774-5.

71. Hommada M, Mekinian A, Brillet PY, et al. Aortitis in giant cell arteritis: diagnosis with FDG PET/CT and agreement with CT angiography. Autoimmun Rev 2017;16(11):1131–7.

72. Berthod PE, Aho-Glélé S, Ornetti P, et al. CT analysis of the aorta in giant-cell arteritis: a case-control study. Eur Radiol 2018;28(9):3676–84.

73. Bienvenu B, Ly KH, Lambert M, et al. Management of giant cell arteritis: recommendations of the French study group for large vessel vasculitis (GEFA). Rev Med Interne 2016;37(3):154–65.

74. Mukhtyar C, Guillevin L, Cid MC, et al. EULAR recommendations for the management of large vessel vasculitis. Ann Rheum Dis 2009;68(3):318–23.

75. Dasgupta B, Borg FA, Hassan N, et al. BSR and BHPR guidelines for the management of giant cell arteritis. Rheumatology 2010;49(8):1594–7.

76. Faurschou M, Ahlström MG, Lindhardsen J, et al. Risk of diabetes mellitus among patients diagnosed with giant cell arteritis or granulomatosis with polyangiitis: comparison with the general population. J Rheumatol 2017;44(1):78–83.

77. de Boysson H, Liozon E, Lambert M, et al. Giant-cell arteritis: do we treat patients with large-vessel involvement differently? Am J Med 2017;130(8):992–5.

78. Nesher G, Nesher R, Mates M, et al. Giant cell arteritis: intensity of the initial systemic inflammatory response and the course of the disease. Clin Exp Rheumatol 2008;26(3 Suppl 49):S30–4.

79. Labarca C, Koster MJ, Crowson CS, et al. Predictors of relapse and treatment outcomes in biopsy-proven giant cell arteritis: a retrospective cohort study. Rheumatology (Oxford) 2016;55(2):347–56.

80. Stone JH, Tuckwell K, Dimonaco S, et al. Glucocorticoid doses and acute-phase reactants at giant cell arteritis flare in a randomized trial of tocilizumab. Arthritis Rheumatol 2019. https://doi.org/10.1002/art.40876.

81. Cheson BD, Fisher RI, Barrington SF, et al. Recommendations for initial evaluation, staging, and response assessment of hodgkin and non-hodgkin lymphoma: the lugano classification. J Clin Oncol 2014;32(27):3059–67.

82. Nielsen BD, Gormsen LC, Hansen IT, et al. Three days of high-dose glucocorticoid treatment attenuates large-vessel 18F-FDG uptake in large-vessel giant cell arteritis but with a limited impact on diagnostic accuracy. Eur J Nucl Med Mol Imaging 2018;45(7):1119–28.

83. Muto G, Yamashita H, Takahashi Y, et al. Large vessel vasculitis in elderly patients: early diagnosis and steroid-response evaluation with FDG-PET/CT and contrast-enhanced CT. Rheumatol Int 2014;1545–54. https://doi.org/10.1007/s00296-014-2985-3.

84. Henes JC, Mueller M, Pfannenberg C, et al. Cyclophosphamide for large vessel vasculitis: assessment of response by PET/CT. Clin Exp Rheumatol 2008;29:S43–8.

85. Grayson PC, Alehashemi S, Bagheri AA, et al. 18 F-Fluorodeoxyglucose-Positron emission tomography as an imaging biomarker in a prospective, longitudinal cohort of patients with large vessel vasculitis. Arthritis Rheumatol 2018;70(3):439–49.

86. Scheel AK, Meller J, Vosshenrich R, et al. Diagnosis and follow up of aortitis in the elderly. Ann Rheum Dis 2004;63(11):1507–10.

87. de Boysson H, Aide N, Liozon E, et al. Repetitive18F-FDG-PET/CT in patients with large-vessel giant-cell arteritis and controlled disease. Eur J Intern Med 2017;46:66–70.

88. Czihal M, Piller A, Schroettle A, et al. Outcome of giant cell arteritis of the arm arteries managed with medical treatment alone: cross-sectional follow-up study. Rheumatology (Oxford) 2013;52(2):282–6.

89. Prieto-González S, García-Martínez A, Tavera-Bahillo I, et al. Effect of glucocorticoid treatment on computed tomography angiography detected large-vessel inflammation in giant-cell arteritis. A prospective, longitudinal study. Medicine (Baltimore) 2015;94(5):e486.

90. de Boysson H, Liozon E, Lambert M, et al. 18F-fluorodeoxyglucose positron emission tomography and the risk of subsequent aortic complications in giant-cell arteritis: a multicenter cohort of 130 patients. Medicine (Baltimore) 2016;95(26):e3851.

91. Banerjee S, Quinn KA, Gribbons KB, et al. Effect of treatment on imaging, clinical, and serologic assessments of disease activity in large-vessel vasculitis. J Rheumatol 2019. https://doi.org/10.3899/jrheum.181222.

Use of ^{18}F-Fluorodeoxyglucose PET in the Diagnosis and Follow-up of Polymyalgia Rheumatica

Albrecht Betrains, MD, Daniel Blockmans, MD, PhD*

KEYWORDS

• FDG • PET • Polymyalgia rheumatica • Large vessel vasculitis • Diagnosis

KEY POINTS

- The diagnosis of polymyalgia rheumatica is usually straightforward based on characteristic clinical findings and increased levels of inflammatory markers, but the symptom complex may be mimicked by many inflammatory and malignant conditions.
- A total skeletal score of greater than or equal to 16, calculated based on ^{18}F- fluorodeoxyglucose (FDG) PET results, has an excellent sensitivity and specificity for polymyalgia rheumatica.
- In patients with polymyalgia rheumatica, FDG-PET may assist in identifying concurrent large vessel vasculitis.
- Cost-effectiveness and clinical utility of FDG-PET should be considered in patients suspected of polymyalgia rheumatica to identify those most likely to derive benefit from this imaging modality.

INTRODUCTION

Polymyalgia rheumatica (PMR) is a common inflammatory disorder in patients more than 50 years of age, characterized by girdle pain in the shoulders and hips, neck pain, morning stiffness, and increased inflammatory parameters. PMR may be found in association with giant cell arteritis (GCA) or rheumatoid arthritis (RA), or as an isolated phenomenon.[1,2] Clinical symptoms often respond promptly to treatment with low-dose glucocorticoids, and this empiric therapeutic strategy is often used as a diagnostic test. Nonetheless, response to glucocorticoids is not specific for PMR and unnecessary treatment should be avoided.

In 2012, provisional classification criteria for PMR were published, based on results from a study in 125 patients with PMR and 169 subjects without PMR.[3] The investigators stated explicitly that these criteria are not intended for diagnostic purposes. Patients could be classified as PMR if they were at least 50 years of age and presenting with bilateral shoulder pain, not better explained by other conditions, in the presence of morning stiffness of at least 45 minutes, increased C-reactive protein (CRP) level and/or erythrocyte sedimentation rate, and new-onset hip pain. The sensitivity (68%) and specificity (78%) of these clinical criteria were limited, and addition of ultrasonography investigation did not significantly improve the sensitivity (66%) or specificity (81%).

The diagnosis of PMR is usually straightforward based on characteristic clinical findings and increased inflammatory markers. Nonetheless,

Funding: None.
Department of General Internal Medicine, University Hospital Gasthuisberg, Herestraat 49, Leuven 3000, Belgium
* Corresponding author.
E-mail address: daniel.blockmans@uzleuven.be

diligence is warranted when atypical symptoms and signs are present or the inflammatory parameters are not as high as expected, considering the symptom complex may be mimicked by many inflammatory and malignant conditions. In the past, this was reflected in the Jones and Hazleman[4] criteria (1981), which required exclusion of RA or other inflammatory arthropathy, myopathy, and malignancy. In those circumstances, additional investigations are advised.

18F-FLUORODEOXYGLUCOSE PET FINDINGS IN POLYMYALGIA RHEUMATICA

PET imaging has contributed significantly to defining PMR as a disease involving (peri)articular and extra-articular structures. In 2007, our group published a prospective study on 35 patients with a clinical diagnosis of PMR, who underwent 18F-fluorodeoxyglucose (FDG) PET at diagnosis (before start of glucocorticoid therapy), and at 3 and 6 months after initiation of treatment.[5] At the time of diagnosis, FDG avidity around the shoulders, hips, and around the spinous processes of the lumbar or cervical vertebrae was noted in 94%, 89%, and 51% of patients, respectively

(Fig. 1A, B). Yamashita and colleagues[6] performed FDG-PET/computed tomography (CT) in 14 patients with untreated, active PMR and 17 control patients with RA or other active rheumatic diseases. They reported similar involvement of the sternoclavicular and shoulder joints in both groups, but a higher frequency of FDG uptake than control patients at the hip joints, ischial tuberosities, greater trochanters, and spinous processes. Rehak and colleagues[7] retrospectively analyzed 67 patients fulfilling the Healey and Sheets[2] criteria for PMR with positive PET/CT results. They detected articular or periarticular involvement in 88.1% and extra-articular involvement (interspinous, ischiogluteal, and prepubic bursae) in 76.1% of patients with PMR, respectively. Publications reporting on multiple sites of FDG accumulation in patients with PMR are summarized in **Table 1**.[5–11]

The exact structures involved in the spine cannot be recognized on PET because of the low spatial resolution of this technique. Based on our findings of increased FDG uptake at the spinous processes, Salvarani and colleagues[12,13] used magnetic resonance imaging to compare patients with PMR versus patients with various other

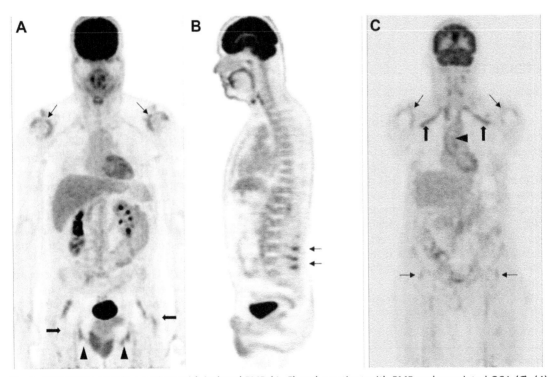

Fig. 1. FDG-PET images in a patient with isolated PMR (A, B) and a patient with PMR and associated GCA (C). (A) Maximum-intensity-projection showing FDG uptake at the shoulders (arrows), hips (block arrows), and bursae around ischial tuberosities (arrowheads). (B) Sagittal image revealing FDG uptake at the cervical and lumbar interspinous processes (arrows). (C) Coronal image showing FDG uptake at the shoulder and hip girdle (arrows) with vasculitis of the subclavian arteries (block arrows) and the ascending aorta (arrowhead).

Table 1
Studies reporting on fluorine-18 fluorodeoxyglucose uptake in different anatomic locations in patients with polymyalgia rheumatica

Publication	Number of Patients	Shoulders	Hips	Sternoclavicular Joint	Ischial Tuberosities	Spinous Processes		Anywhere	Symphysis	Subtrochanteric Bursae	Vasculitis
						Cervical	Lumbar				
Blockmans et al,[5] 2007	35	33 (94)	31 (85)	—	—	—	—	18 (51)	—	—	11 (31)
Yamashita et al,[6] 2012	14	12 (86)	12 (86)	6 (43)	12 (86)	1 (7)	11 (79)	11 (79)	—	10 (71)	9 (64)
Rehak et al,[7] 2015	67	58 (87)	47 (70)	31 (46)	35 (52)	13 (19)	38 (57)	—	5 (8)	—	27 (40)
Palard-Novello et al,[8] 2016	18	16 (89)	17 (94)	13 (72)	17 (94)	10 (56)	13 (72)	—	—	—	0 (0)
Wakura et al,[11] 2016	15	12 (80)	11 (73)	9 (60)	14 (93)	7 (47)	11 (73)	—	9 (60)	14 (93)	—
Rehak et al,[9] 2017	15	15 (100)	15 (100)	14 (93)	14 (93)	4 (27)	13 (87)	14 (93)	15 (100)	—	5 (33)
Henckaerts et al,[10] 2018	67	67 (100)	61 (91)	57 (85)	64 (95)	60 (90)	56 (83)	—	—	66 (99)	12 (15)

inflammatory and noninflammatory causes of spinal pain. They identified interspinal bursitis of the cervical and lumbar spine as the typical alteration in patients with PMR. In contrast with ultrasonography, PET may allow assessment of deep bursae such as spinous processes, ischial tuberosities, and greater trochanters.

The specificity of these PET findings for PMR remained unclear. However, in 2018, the authors published a prospective study on 99 patients with a possible clinical diagnosis of PMR who underwent FDG-PET scanning before initiation of glucocorticoid treatment.[10] We quantified the clinical suspicion (range, 1–5) of PMR and visually scored the FDG uptake in 12 articular regions (shoulders, hips, sternoclavicular joints, ischial tuberosities, greater trochanters, cervical spinous processes, and lumbar spinous processes). A total skeletal score was calculated, reflecting FDG uptake (range, 0–2) in these regions. Sixty-seven patients were diagnosed with PMR, whereas 32 patients got an alternative diagnosis. The gold standard for a diagnosis of PMR was the judgment of an experienced clinician after at least 6 months of follow-up, taking into account all available information (clinical data and evolution, biochemical and technical data). **Table 2** shows the sensitivity, specificity, positive predictive value, and negative predictive value of the clinical score and the total skeletal score.

The authors acknowledge this study had some limitations, as was also stated by Clifford and Cimmino.[14] The gold standard diagnosis was made, including the results of the test under evaluation, introducing the problem of circular reasoning. However, because of the lack of a true gold standard for the diagnosis of PMR and the limited sensitivity of the classification criteria, we consider our approach to be appropriate.

Table 2
Sensitivity, specificity, positive predictive value, and negative predictive value of clinical score and total skeletal score in patients with polymyalgia rheumatica

	Sensitivity (%)	Specificity (%)	PPV (%)	NPV (%)
Clinical Score ≥4	67.2	87.5	91.8	56.0
Total Skeletal Score ≥16	85.1	87.5	93.4	73.7

Abbreviations: NPV, negative predictive value; PPV, positive predictive value.

An additional advantage of FDG-PET in the diagnostic work-up of patients suspected of PMR may be the exclusion of other disorders, especially malignancies and other inflammatory conditions that can present with a PMR-like picture. In our patient group without PMR, 1 patient was diagnosed with a carcinoid neoplasm, which was visualized on FDG-PET, and symptoms could be explained as paraneoplastic manifestations.

ROLE OF ^{18}F-FLUORODEOXYGLUCOSE PET IN THE FOLLOW-UP OF POLYMYALGIA RHEUMATICA

In our earlier mentioned prospective study on 35 patients with a clinical diagnosis of PMR, FDG-PET was repeated at 3 and 6 months after initiation of glucocorticoid therapy.[5] Repetitive FDG-PET after 3 months of glucocorticoid treatment resulted in a decrease of FDG uptake in shoulders, hips, and spinous processes. At 3 months, all but 2 patients who had relapsed around that time were asymptomatic, and laboratory parameters of inflammation had significantly decreased. The decrease in FDG uptake is presumably consistent with a lower disease activity. However, sedimentation rate and CRP levels reflect the same and are much cheaper to perform. Accordingly, repetitive FDG-PET imaging is not justified to assess treatment response.

Compared with patients without relapse, patients who relapsed had similar FDG uptake in large joints and spinous processes at baseline and after 3 months of treatment. Consequently, we could not conclude that patients with persistent articular FDG accumulation at 3 months were more prone to relapse in the months to come.

ROLE OF ^{18}F-FLUORODEOXYGLUCOSE PET IN ASSESSING LARGE VESSEL VASCULITIS IN POLYMYALGIA RHEUMATICA

GCA occurs in up to 21% of patients with PMR, and approximately 50% of patients with GCA present with PMR before, at the time of, or after the diagnosis of vasculitis.[1,15] Furthermore, GCA may relapse as PMR or vice versa. PET may contribute to identifying large vessel vasculitis associated with PMR. The authors showed increased vascular FDG uptake, predominantly in the subclavian arteries, in one-third of 35 patients with isolated PMR (**Fig. 1**C).[5] However, compared with GCA, the intensity of the FDG uptake was less marked, with only 2 out of 35 patients showing intense vascular FDG accumulation. Yamashita and colleagues[6] identified increased vascular FDG uptake in only 2 out of 14 untreated patients with PMR. Prieto-Peña and colleagues[16] analyzed 51 patients with evidence of large vessel vasculitis on FDG-PET in a group of 84 patients with classic PMR symptoms. The reasons to perform an FDG-PET scan were persistence of classic PMR symptoms despite glucocorticoid treatment, occurrence of unusual manifestations, marked constitutional symptoms, and unexplained increase in levels of acute phase proteins despite glucocorticoid treatment. Patients with evidence of large vessel vasculitis on PET-CT often had unusual PMR symptoms, including inflammatory lower back pain and diffuse lower limb pain. Their results showed that bilateral diffuse lower limb pain, pelvic girdle pain, and inflammatory lower back pain were statistically significant predictors for the presence of large vessel vasculitis on PET-CT scan. The investigators mentioned some limitations of this study, including the absence of histologic confirmation of large vessel vasculitis and active treatment with glucocorticoids at the time of FDG-PET assessment.

ROLE OF ^{18}F-FLUORODEOXYGLUCOSE PET IN THE DIFFERENTIAL DIAGNOSIS OF POLYMYALGIA RHEUMATICA AND RHEUMATOID ARTHRITIS

In terms of differential diagnosis, FDG-PET may be useful in distinguishing PMR as an isolated phenomenon from PMR occurring in the context of RA. Some investigators evaluated FDG uptake in patients with PMR compared with RA. Yamashita and colleagues[6] compared FDG uptake at different anatomic locations in 27 patients with PMR with 10 patients with elderly onset RA. Although FDG accumulation of the periarticular structures of the shoulder had a similar prevalence in both groups, abnormal uptake at the ischial tuberosity, spinous processes, and iliopectineal bursa was significantly higher in PMR compared with RA. Wakura and colleagues[11] compared abnormal FDG uptake sites between 15 patients with PMR and 7 patients with elderly onset RA in whom PET/CT was performed. They reported significantly higher FDG uptake at the enthesis of the pectineus and rectus femoris muscle, the scapulohumeral joint, the lateral side of the greater trochanter, the ischial tuberosity, hip joint, spinous process of the cervical and lumbar vertebra, and intervertebral joint of the lumbar vertebra in the PMR group compared with the elderly onset RA group. They suggested PET/CT may be useful for differentiating PMR from elderly onset RA.

SUMMARY

FDG-PET is not required for the diagnosis of PMR in patients presenting with a typical clinical picture. However, atypical presentations occur and may indicate an underlying disorder. Consideration of cost-effectiveness and clinical utility of FDG-PET is warranted to identify patients with PMR most likely to derive benefit from this imaging modality. A total skeletal score of greater than or equal to 16, calculated based on FDG-PET results, has an excellent sensitivity (85.1%) and specificity (87.5%) for PMR. Furthermore, FDG-PET may assist in identifying patients with concurrent large vessel vasculitis and patients with a PMR-like picture occurring in the context of other inflammatory conditions or malignancies.

DISCLOSURE

The authors have no conflicts of interest. There is no relevant information to disclose.

REFERENCES

1. Weyand C, Goronzy J. Giant-cell arteritis and polymyalgia rheumatica. N Engl J Med 2014;371(1): 50–7.
2. Healey L, Sheets P. The relation of polymyalgia rheumatica to rheumatoid arthritis. J Rheumatol 1988; 15(5):750–2.
3. Dasgupta B, Cimmino M, Salvarani C, et al. 2012 provisional classification criteria for polymyalgia rheumatica: a European League against Rheumatism/American College of Rheumatology. Arthritis Rheum 2012;64(4):943–54.
4. Jones JG, Hazleman BL. Polymyalgia rheumatica and giant cell arteritis—a difficult diagnosis. JR Coll Gen Pract 1981;31(226):283–9.
5. Blockmans D, De Ceuninck L, Bobbaers H, et al. Repetitive 18-fluorodeoxyglucose positron emission tomography in isolated polymyalgia rheumatica: a prospective study in 35 patients. Rheumatology 2006;46(4):672–7.
6. Yamashita H, Kubota K, Ito K, et al. Whole-body fluorodeoxyglucose positron emission tomography/computed tomography in patients with active polymyalgia rheumatica: evidence for distinctive bursitis and large-vessel vasculitis. Mod Rheumatol 2012; 22(5):705–11.
7. Rehak Z, Vasina J, Bortlicek Z, et al. Various forms of 18F-FDG PET and PET/CT findings in patients with polymyalgia rheumatica. Biomed Pap Med Fac Univ Palacky Olomouc Czech Repub 2015;159(4): 629–36.
8. Palard-Novello X, Querellou S, Garrigues F, et al. Value of 18 F-FDG PET/CT for therapeutic assessment of patients with polymyalgia rheumatica

receiving tocilizumab as first-line treatment. Eur J Nucl Med Mol Imaging 2016;43(4):773–9.

9. Rehak Z, Sprlakova-Pukova A, Joukal M, et al. PET/CT imaging in polymyalgia rheumatica: praepubic 18F-FDG uptake correlates with pectineus and adductor longus muscles enthesitis and with tenosynovitis. Radiol Oncol 2017;51(1):8–14.

10. Henckaerts L, Gheysens O, Blockmans D. Use of 18F-fluorodeoxyglucose positron emission tomography in the diagnosis of polymyalgia rheumatica—a prospective study of 99 patients. Rheumatology 2017;57(11):1908–16.

11. Wakura D, Kotani T, Makino S, et al. Differentiation between polymyalgia rheumatica (PMR) and elderly-onset rheumatoid arthritis using 18F-fluorodeoxyglucose positron emission tomography/computed tomography: is enthesitis a new pathological lesion in PMR? PLoS One 2016;11(7): e0158509.

12. Salvarani C, Barozzi L, Alentino M, et al. Cervical interspinous bursitis in active polymyalgia rheumatica. Ann Rheum Dis 2008;67(6):758–61.

13. Salvarani C, Barozzi L, Macchioni P, et al. Lumbar interspinous bursitis in active polymyalgia rheumatica. Clin Exp Rheumatol 2013;31(4):526–31.

14. Clifford A, Cimmino M. In search of a diagnostic test for polymyalgia rheumatica: is positron emission tomography the answer? Rheumatology 2018;57:1881–2.

15. Salvarani C, Cantini F, Hunder G. Polymyalgia rheumatica and giant-cell arteritis. N Engl J Med 2002; 347(4):261–71.

16. Prieto-Peña D, Martínez-Rodríguez I, Calvo-Río V, et al. Predictors of positive 18F-FDG PET/CT-scan for large vessel vasculitis in patients with persistent polymyalgia rheumatica. Semin Arthritis Rheum 2019;48(4):720–7.

FDG-PET/CT in Inflammatory Bowel Disease: Is There a Future?

Jacob Broder Brodersen, MD[a], Søren Hess, MD[b,c],*

KEYWORDS

- Inflammatory bowel disease • Ulcerative colitis • Crohn disease • PET • Computed tomography
- PET/CT • FDG • MR imaging

KEY POINTS

- Fluorodeoxyglucose (FDG)-PET/computed tomography (CT) has shown promise in inflammatory bowel disease with generally good sensitivity and specificity in various settings, but its overall role is controversial.
- Many issues remain unresolved, and there is no consensus on imaging protocol in the literature. More studies with stringent methodology are needed.
- Combining FDG-PET with CT or MR enterography yields more information than either examination alone.
- At present, the most promising roles are assessment of early treatment response and stricture characterization, whereas general use in the initial diagnostic workup should be reserved for equivocal cases.

INTRODUCTION

Crohn disease (CD) and ulcerative colitis (UC) belong to the group of chronic inflammatory bowel diseases (IBDs). The cause is unknown, but is thought to arise from a dysregulated interaction between the gut microbiome and the mucosal immune system in a genetically predisposed individual.[1]

In CD, the inflammation is transmural and granulomatous; the distribution is typically segmental, and the entire gastrointestinal tract may be involved, from mouth to anus. Most frequently, the disease is located at the terminal ileum and right colon (ileocecal CD). In approximately one-third of patients, the disease is located at the small

intestine, and one-third of patients have CD restricted to the colon.[2]

In contrast to CD, UC is restricted to the colon; the inflammation extends from the rectum, and the inflammation is submucosal and nongranulomatous.

Clinically, CD and UC are both characterized by recurrent disease activity, and a strong tendency to relapse after remission has been achieved with medical treatment or surgical resection. A small proportion of patients experiences continuous disease activity.[3] Current guidelines for diagnosing CD and UC suggest ileocolonoscopy with multiple biopsies from the terminal ileum and each colonic segment as the first diagnostic examination.[4] However, in the case of CD, irrespective of the findings

[a] Department of Gastroenterology, Hospital of Southwest Jutland, Finsensgade 35, Esbjerg Dk-6700, Denmark;
[b] Department of Radiology and Nuclear Medicine, Hospital of Southwest Jutland, Finsensgade 35, Esbjerg Dk-6700, Denmark; [c] Department of Regional Health Research, University of Southern Denmark, Odense, Denmark
* Corresponding author. Department of Radiology and Nuclear Medicine, Hospital of Southwest Jutland, Finsensgade 35, Esbjerg Dk-6700, Denmark.
E-mail address: Soren.hess@rsyd.dk

PET Clin 15 (2020) 153–162
https://doi.org/10.1016/j.cpet.2019.11.006
1556-8598/20/© 2019 Elsevier Inc. All rights reserved.

at ileocolonoscopy, further investigations are recommended to establish the location and extent of any CD in the upper small bowel. Furthermore, the disease pattern of recurrence and relapse as well as the assessment of treatment response necessitates repeated examinations.

Ileocolonoscopy is regarded as the gold standard for diagnosing CD located in the colon and terminal ileum.[5] However, the examination is invasive and is associated with patient discomfort and a small risk of colonic perforation. Furthermore, a complete ileocolonoscopy is not always possible.[5] Thus, the need for noninvasive, patient-friendly, and reliable examinations is in great demand. In recent years, technological advances have improved noninvasive modalities, especially for diagnosing CD. The main modalities are MR imaging, computed tomography (CT), ultrasound, and capsule endoscopy. The latter modalities have all been shown in numerous studies to have a rather good sensitivity and specificity in terms of finding Crohn lesions in the small bowel.[6,7] The latter cross-sectional modalities are rather good, but they are not perfect, and their results are primarily founded on structural changes, although contrast enhancement, Doppler measurements, and diffusion-weighted MR imaging give some clues about vascular status, and thereby, an indirect sign of inflammation.

PET using the radioactive glucose analogue 18F-fluorodeoxyglucose (FDG-PET) has been available for decades, and because it has been combined with CT or MR imaging, it is nowadays a very well-established tool in many fields, especially oncology. In IBD, it is not yet a well-established procedure, and in the recent European guidelines, FDG-PET is not recommended for diagnostics in IBD because of a lack of evidence.[8] However, unlike the structural/anatomic examinations (CT, MR imaging, bowel ultrasound, and capsule endoscopy), FDG-PET is a functional test of metabolic activity. Combining FDG-PET with either CT or MR imaging produces a noninvasive imaging modality combining a metabolic assessment of pathophysiologic processes with precise morphologic correlation. This combination has been shown to be useful in IBD diagnostics.

The purpose of this review is to present the current status on the use of FDG-PET/CT in IBD based on the available literature.

OPTIMIZING THE SCAN

Besides the general issues with 4 to 6 hours of fasting and refraining from strenuous physical activity for 24 hours before the examination, there is no definite consensus on patient preparation before FDG-PET of the bowel; the different studies used different protocols, which to a high degree was dependent on whether FDG-PET was combined with CT or MR imaging. Several factors need to be addressed: among others, peristalsis, indigenous bacterial flora, and active mucosal lining can all result in increased physiologic FDG uptake that may hamper visual interpretation and potentially lead to inaccurate recording of standardized uptake value (SUV) measurements. Toriihara and colleagues[9] highlighted this issue as a possible confounder of bowel activity in a dual time-point imaging study of 61 participants without known bowel disease. They focused on colon segments with visually increased uptake (ie, uptake higher than the liver) and found this in 34 of 156 segments (21%) with mean SUV_{max} of 3.11 in early images and 3.74 in late images.

One possible way to reduce intense physiologic bowel uptake arising from peristalsis is administration of the antispasmodic drug N-butylscopolamine (ie, hyoscinebutylbromide), a drug commonly used in radiology to reduce motion artifacts of the bowel during MR imaging.[10] In a study from 2008, Emmott and colleagues[11] improved accuracy of FDG-PET reporting by significantly reducing artifacts in the bowel during FDG-PET by injection of 20 mg hyoscinebutylbromide 1 minute before FDG administration, whereas Miraldi and colleagues[12] reduced artifacts through colon cleansing with an isosmotic solution taken the evening before examination.

Some protocols suggest improving interpretation by optimizing bowel distention, for example, water as a negative CT negative contrast agent,[13] or mannitol, as in most MR imaging examinations.[14] Zhang and colleagues[15] found oral negative contrast agent and hypotonic bowel preparation decreased the physiologic intake of FDG and increased the distention of the gastrointestinal tract with an overall improvement of image quality.

Finally, it is well known that the widely used antidiabetic metformin may diffusely increase FDG uptake in the small bowel and colon, albeit through unknown mechanisms. The effect is significantly reduced if the drug is stopped for 3 to 5 days before the examination.[16]

PET PERFORMANCE

FDG has been available for more than 40 years,[17] and combined with PET has become part of the recommended diagnostic workup strategy in most malignant diseases and dementia over the last 2 decades.[18] Routine application has also increased within the field of infectious and inflammatory diseases, especially in whole-body ailments like fever of unknown origin and large-vessel vasculitis.[19] The use of FDG in IBD is, however, not as well founded. Although the first case report on the subject was published more than 20 years ago,[20] the evidence and potential role of FDG-PET and FDG-PET/CT in IBD remain controversial.

In terms of diagnostics in IBD, an important distinction is between primary diagnosis and monitoring disease activity; some studies are available on primary diagnosis in patients with suspected IBD, but the main focus in the literature is on monitoring because the abovementioned physiologic uptake may conceal true positive lesions as well as give rise to false-positive findings. Also, because the final diagnosis is based on histopathology, endoscopy is required anyway. It would, however, be desirable with a noninvasive imaging method with a more physiologic approach as an adjunct to the mainstay morphologic modalities for surveillance purposes.

FDG-PET and FDG-PET/CT in Patients Suspected of Inflammatory Bowel Disease

In 1997, Bicik and colleagues[20] reported on the use of FDG-PET in 7 patients with suspected IBD using endoscopy and histology as the gold standard. They showed high PET activity in areas with macroscopic disease as well as in areas of active inflammation on biopsy scan in the absence of macroscopic disease in 6 of 7 patients (2 UC and 4 CD). The investigators concluded that FDG-PET might be a useful tool as a noninvasive means to identify active inflammation in IBD.

Perhaps not surprising, the potential of FDG-PET as a noninvasive primary diagnostic has been explored in pediatric settings. In 1999, Skehan and colleagues[21] reported the use of FDG-PET in 25 pediatric patients (mean age 13) with suspected IBD; colonoscopy and/or small bowel series was the gold standard. A total of 18 patients were identified with IBD: 15 with CD and 3 with UC. FDG-PET correctly identified 60 of 79 (76%) possible regions with sensitivity for identifying inflammation of 71% and a specificity of 81%, whereas the overall patient-based values were 81% and 85%, respectively. The investigators concluded that FDG-PET could be a useful adjunct if conventional studies are technically unsuccessful. However, in a significant proportion of patients, colonoscopies were incomplete, and PET detected more proximal lesions in 80% of

patients. A retrospective study from 2006 by Loeffler and colleagues[22] included 23 pediatric patients with suspected IBD of which 17 cases had CD and 2 cases had UC as the final diagnosis. Of the 23 patients, 18 had a corresponding colonoscopy within 10 days of the FDG-PET, albeit no colonoscopy completion rate or inclusion criteria were reported. The overall sensitivity of FDG-PET was 98% (57/58), and the specificity was 68% (40/59) when compared with histology. When compared with endoscopy, there was a sensitivity of 90% and a specificity of 75%. The investigators reported the FDG-PET was even more accurate in the small intestine.

In 2007, Das and colleagues[23] made an effort to improve the CT part of the FDG-PET/CT by combining PET with CT enteroclysis. Of the 17 patients included in the study, 15 had an ileocolonoscopy, and all had other radiologic evaluation as per standard of care, that is, the gold standard was endoscopy, radiology, or both. The final diagnoses included CD (n = 9), intestinal tuberculosis (n = 5), tropical sprue (n = 2), and celiac disease (n = 1), and no subgroup analyses were performed with CD alone. They concluded that FDG-PET/CT enteroclysis as a single investigation detects a significantly higher number of lesions in both the small and large intestine in comparison to that detected by conventional barium and colonoscopy combined. Also, this was the first study to report extraintestinal findings (ie, sacroiliitis and lymphadenopathy) and suggest this to be a potential advantage of whole-body FDG-PET/CT over conventional imaging.

FDG-PET and FDG-PET/CT in Patients with Known Inflammatory Bowel Disease

Whereas the evidence for the use of FDG-PET or FDG-PET/CT in the primary diagnostic setting is rather scarce, the use in patients with known disease is better studied. Again, the early studies were with stand-alone PET.

Starting in 2002, Neurath and colleagues[24] studied the use of FDG-PET in a prospective setup, with 59 (+12 controls) patients with chronic active CD, using colonoscopy (28/59), MR imaging, or antigranulocyte scintigraphy in comparisons. For the detection of inflamed segments of the small and large bowel segments, PET was found to have a sensitivity of 85%, higher than hydro-MR imaging (41%) and antigranulocyte scintigraphy (67%), with a specificity of 89% compared with 93% and 100% for hydro-MR imaging and antigranulocyte scintigraphy, respectively. Neurath and colleagues[24] concluded that FDG-PET appeared to be a reliable noninvasive tool for simultaneous detection of inflamed areas in the small and large bowel of patients with CD. It is, however, worth considering that sensitivity and specificity of FDG-PET was based only on data from the 28 patients with colonoscopy (45% of included patients), and 24 of 127 lesions detected with PET were actually in areas inaccessible to endoscopy and thus not further classified.

In 2005, Lemberg and colleagues[25] enrolled 65 children in the first and to date only prospective case-control study: 55 children (aged 7–18 years) with newly diagnosed IBD (n = 37) or symptoms suggestive of recurrent disease (n = 18), and as controls, 10 children with recurrent abdominal pain (aged 8–15 years). All had FDG-PET scans, and the results were compared with small bowel follow-through with pneumocolon and/or colonoscopy. They found 38 patients had CD and 17 had UC. In patients with CD, compared with colonoscopy, FDG-PET correctly identified the presence of inflammation in 1 segment in 90% of cases with a specificity of 50%, although the study was limited by the poor intubation rate of the terminal ileum. In the patients with UC, FDG-PET identified inflammation correctly in at least 1 bowel segment in 14 of 17 cases leading to a sensitivity of 81% when compared with colonoscopy. Furthermore, FDG-PET was correct without evidence of inflammation in children with recurrent abdominal pain. Lemberg and colleagues concluded that FDG-PET may not be able to replace conventional studies, but is a noninvasive tool for identifying and localizing active intestinal inflammation in children with IBD. However, several caveats pertain to this study: Several issues may have contributed to the rather poor sensitivity, for example, a gap between FDG-PET and reference standards of as much as 62 days together with anti-inflammatory treatment being initiated may have inadvertently led to false negative findings. Furthermore, 3 fibrotic stenoses not detected by FDG-PET were also considered false negative, although FDG is not taken up by metabolically inert fibrosis in contrast to inflammatory stricture. On the other hand, colonoscopies were only sufficient in half of the patients, and inflammatory lesions proximal to the colonoscopies were classified as false positive, which may have contributed to the poor specificity.

Hybrid-PET/CT

The introduction of combined hybrid PET/CT opened up new possibilities, and in 2007, 2 such studies were published. One included both UC and CD; the other only CD. Both were compared with colonoscopy. In the study by Meisner and colleagues,[26] FDG activity was seen in 13 of 24 (52%)

regions in patients with UC and 19 of 32 (59.4%) regions in patients with CD. There was a high correlation between FDG activity and disease activity as determined by colonoscopy, disease activity indices, and radiology (in UC 23 of 24 [96%]; in CD 26 of 32 [81%]). It is worth mentioning, though, that FDG-PET/CT only assessed the ileocolonic area, although CD may affect the entire gastrointestinal tract. In the study by Louis and colleagues,[13] 22 patients with active CD were included. All had colonoscopy, although in 5 cases strictures caused the colonoscopy to be incomplete. A total of 48 lesions were found at colonoscopy, whereas FDG-PET/CT found 35 of the affected segments, leading to a sensitivity and specificity of 73% and 55%, respectively, in terms of finding endoscopic visible lesions. They found sensitivity to be improved in cases with severe endoscopic lesion. Also, CT found signs of inflammation in PET-positive areas not detected by endoscopy, which raises the possibility that the poor specificity owing to false-positive scans may be incorrectly low if some of these lesions were in fact true positives.

The focus on optimizing scan and the value of combining FDG-PET with CT was investigated by several groups in 2010. Groshar and colleagues[27] published the use of FDG-PET and CT enterography (CTE) in 28 patients with known or suspected CD. They found good correlation between SUV_{max} and mural thickness and a significant difference between SUV_{max} in normal versus abnormal segments. The study also illustrated the challenge with colonoscopy: 63% of patients with a normal colonoscopy exhibited abnormal segments on CTE.

In a retrospective study, Ahmadi and colleagues[28] evaluated 41 FDG-PET/CTE scans of patients with known CD. Here, 38 of 48 abnormal bowel segments on CTE had increased FDG uptake. FDG-PET did not identify additional segments not identified by CTE, but abnormal segments on CTE without increased FDG uptake were associated with failure of medical therapy (P = .001); hence, the investigators conclude that this might help identify patients at high risk of failing medical treatment.

In a prospective study by Shyn and colleagues[29] with 13 known CD patients, CTE and FDG-PET/CTE were compared, using endoscopy (n = 7) or surgery (n = 6) as reference. The combined FDG-PET/CTE did not detect diseased bowel segments that were not already evident on CTE alone. CTE alone and combined PET/CTE both detected 100% of bowel segments with more than mild disease activity; the specificity was 90%. Thus, FDG was better at detecting moderate to severe lesions than mild lesions. The combined scan also discovered an enterocolic fistula that otherwise would have been missed.

In a publication from Das and colleagues,[30] FDG-PET was combined with CT-colonography in 15 patients with active UC using colonoscopy as reference standard. There was a good correlation between SUV_{max} and endoscopic activity level when compared ($\kappa = 55.3\%$, $P = .02$). Six patients had a one-to-one correlation between FDG uptake scores and endoscopy activity grades, and in 7 patients, FDG-PET/CT revealed extraintestinal findings. The investigators did not elaborate on colonoscopy success rate, and incomplete colonoscopy could explain the discrepancies.

Finally, Holtmann and colleagues[31] compared FDG-PET to MR imaging in 43 patients using colonoscopy as a reference standard. In a total of 241 segments, 80 showed endoscopic activity, and 72 (sensitivity 90% and specificity 93%) and 53 (sensitivity 66% and specificity 99%) were detected by FDG-PET and MR imaging, respectively. In 2012, Treglia and colleagues[32] published a metaanalysis of 7 studies enrolling a total of 219 patients. They found a pooled per-segment sensitivity of 85% and specificity of 87%.

Strictures

One of the troublesome issues when treating patients with CD is obstructive disease, because strictures that are primarily of inflammatory in nature can be treated with medicine, whereas primarily fibrotic strictures are only treatable with surgery. Several studies have tried to use FDG-PET or FDG-PET/CT to establish the underlying cause of strictures in order to predict the right treatment strategy. Thus, the abovementioned study by Holtmann also focused on stenosis in a subset of patients; they used stand-alone PET only, but confirmed inflammation in 16 of 17 stenoses with 1 false-negative finding.[31]

Jacene and colleagues[33] tried predicting the need for surgical intervention in obstructive CD by FDG-PET/CT in 17 patients scheduled to undergo surgical resection because of obstructive symptoms. Twelve of 13 patients who underwent surgery had pathologic correlation with the predominant histopathologies being inflammation (n = 5), fibrosis (n = 4), and muscle hypertrophy (n = 3), but in all patients, there was significant overlap of the histologic features. Of the 12 patients, 10 were considered to have active inflammation by visual assessment of FDG-PET/CT. When a cutoff value was applied to maximum standardized uptake value corrected for lean body mass (SUL_{max}), a value of greater than 8 predicted inflammation with a sensitivity of 60% and a specificity of 100%. SUL_{max} was also significantly higher in severe versus mild to moderate inflammation, and no patient with predominantly fibrotic or muscle hypertrophic stenosis has SUL_{max} values greater than 8. The investigators concluded that stenosis in CD usually comprise a continuum of inflammation, fibrosis, and muscle hypertrophy, and although FDG-PET/CT could not consistently differentiate between active inflammation, fibrotic stricture, and muscular hypertrophy, it may help clinicians decide on treatment strategy with the combination of visual/qualitative and semiquantitative assessment.

In a prospective setting, Lenze and colleagues[34] compared the diagnostic accuracy of MR imaging, FDG-PET/CT, and ultrasound. No single modality was superior compared with the others for detection and differentiation of strictures in 30 CD patients with 37 CD-associated strictures (22 inflamed, 12 mixed, and 3 fibrostenotic), but a combined diagnostic approach using FDG-PET/CT or MR enterography (MR-E) combined with ultrasound resulted in a 100% detection rate of symptomatic strictures requiring interventions. However, there were only 3 patients with fibromatous strictures in the study, and the gold standard was an unvalidated scoring system combining endoscopy and histology rather than surgical specimen, as in other studies.

Response evaluation

A functional test of metabolic activity FDG-PET/CT may help predict response to treatment faster and more reliably that conventional cross-sectional imaging.

In 2010, Spier and colleagues[35] conducted a small pilot study on 5 IBD patients (3 CD and 2 UC) with FDG-PET/CT before and after treatment. Each patient had 5 bowel segments scored (0–3) for FDG uptake with the liver as reference. After an average of 437 days (range 77–807), the posttreatment PET/CT scan was performed. All patients showed significantly improved physician global assessment scores ($P = .004$). The total PET score of all segments was 32 pretreatment and 14 posttreatment ($P<.01$). Of 11 pretreatment active segments, 9 (82%) segments became either inactive or displayed decreased activity, whereas 2 showed no change ($P<.001$). The investigators concluded that FDG-PET/CT score decreased with successful treatment of inflammation in active IBD and correlated with symptom improvement. However, several severe caveats pertain to the study: the study included only patients with colonic disease; treatment regimens differed; and the gap between pretreatment and posttreatment scan was long and highly variable.

In 2016, Russo and colleagues[36] assessed the utility of FDG-PET/CT as a marker of progression of inflammatory activity and its response to treatment in patients with CD. Twenty-two patients with known active CD and scheduled to start anti–tumor necrosis factor alpha (TNF-α) treatment were recruited prospectively to undergo FDG-PET/CT scanning pretreatment and 12 weeks posttreatment. All 22 patients' index scans were used to assess sensitivity and specificity against a reference standard MR imaging measure (Ma-RIA). The sensitivity and specificity of FDG-PET/CT were 88% and 70%, respectively, which correlated well with previous studies. Of the 22 patients included, 17 completed the posttreatment scan, and SUV-based PET results correlated significantly with C-reactive protein and Harvey-Bradshaw Index in cross-sectional and longitudinal analyses. There were significant differences in clinical responders compared with nonresponders in terms of reduction in SUV-related measures. Surprisingly, there were very poor correlations to fecal calprotectin, which is one of the standard tools in the follow-up of CD patients. The investigators concluded FDG-PET/CT might be useful for longitudinal monitoring of inflammatory activity in CD.

In 2017, Epelboym and colleagues[37] studied the possibility of using FDG-PET/CT to predict treatment response to anti-TNF-α treatment in 8 patients with known CD. All patients had clinically active CD and were planned to start biologic treatment. An index FDG-PET/CT was performed within a week before the first dose of anti-TNF-α, and the second scan was performed after 2 weeks before the second dose of anti-TNF-α. A positive-response scan was characterized as one with at least 30% decrease of FDG activity in the most FDG-avid bowel loop. Of 8 enrolled patients, 7 displayed a decline in FDG avidity at 2 weeks. Five of them were determined to have a clinical response and to be in steroid-free remission at weeks 8, 26, and 52. However, 2 of the 7 patients with reduced FDG activity were determined to not have a clinical response but did display an interval decline in the biochemical inflammatory marker CRP at 8 weeks. One patient with no decrease in FDG avidity did not display any clinical or biochemical response, and no steroid-free remission at any follow-up time points of anti-TNF-α therapy following the first FDG-PET/CT. The study was limited by size, but it did show FDG-PET/CT has the potential to monitor early treatment response and predict clinical response in patients with active CD before a second dose of anti-TNF therapy. Further and larger studies are needed to make firmer conclusions on whether a lack of PET response before

second dose predicts anti-TNF-α failure in patients with CD.

In 2017, Palatka and colleagues[38] used FDG-PET/CT to evaluate treatment response in 12 CD patients before and 1 year after anti-TNF-α treatment. All patients had colonoscopy as a reference. They describe a clearly visible difference in terms of inflammatory sites on PET/CT. However, changes in the global PET score used to express activity of CD as a single number was not significantly different in various settings, except in a subgroup of patients with a high initial score. In clinical and endoscopic scores, the change was significant. Results corresponded to other studies whereby high initial activity on FDG-PET or FDG-PET/CT was a predictor of response. In this setup, the use of the PET score was questionable because it only showed significant results in the subgroup with the most severe baseline inflammation, but the study was limited in size.

Novel Approaches: Quantification and PET/MR Imaging

Despite the widespread acceptance of SUV-based parameters also among clinicians, it is well known to the nuclear medicine community that this methodology has its shortcomings; standardized protocols are pivotal to reduce the many potential pitfalls both technical and patient related, and to this effect novel quantification methods are being explored.[39]

In a publication from 2014, data from a prior prospective study were used to test the feasibility of novel volume-based quantification methods to measure more globally the degree of inflammation in CD based on FDG-PET/CT. To access global inflammation, all pathologic lesions have to be summed up in a single number and preferentially so by using partial volume corrected (PVC) value of total glycolysis in all lesions (ie, total lesion glycolysis; TLG) by summing mean values of SUV. Thus, a global CD activity score (GCDAS) was calculated as the sum of PVC-TLG over all clinically significant FDG-avid regions in each subject. GCDAS significantly correlated with Crohn's Disease Activity Index and fecal calprotectin ($r = 0.64$ and $r = 0.51$, respectively; $P<.05$).[40] A drawback to this method is that it is time consuming and requires strictly standardized protocols.

Berry and colleagues[41] showed in a study of 60 patients with known UC the correlation between MAYO score and FDG uptake. Rectal PET activity showed a significant correlation with the Mayo score ($k = 0.465$, $P<.001$), endoscopic subscore ($k = 0.526$, $P<.001$), histologic score ($k = 0.496$,

$P<.001$), and fecal calprotectin (k = 0.279, $P = .031$). Extent evaluation by FDG-PET/CT and colonoscopy showed a significant correlation (k = 0.582, $P<.001$).

Over the past few years, attention has turned to the possible role of FDG-PET/MR imaging scanners, which have the potential to not only combine the good image qualities of MR imaging, a well-known tool in IBD, with the functional component of FDG-PET, but also reduce the radioactive burden. In a prospective pilot study enrolling 21 patients with known CD, Domachevsky and colleagues[42] found that adding apparent diffusion coefficient and metabolic inflammatory volume to MaRIA score resulted in an area under the curve (AUC) of 0.92 (compared with MaRIA alone with an AUC of 0.63), resulting in 83% sensitivity and 100% specificity.

In another study on FDG-PET/MR imaging in 50 patients with known CD, Li and colleagues[43] showed wall thickness and the comb sign to be the most important parameters for detecting segments with active inflammation of any type. In terms of quantification, SUV_{max} ratio from PET was the most important parameter for detecting severely inflamed segments with ulceration. Finally, in a recent paper, Li and colleagues[44] introduced an FDG-PET/MR imaging index defined as (0.87 × wall thickness) + (1.97 × edema) + (0.83 × ulceration) + (0.55 × SUV_{max} ratio) + 1.14. When FDG-PET/MR imaging index was compared with MaRIA score, sensitivity was comparable (0.855 vs 0.894, $P>.05$), but specificity was better with the FDG-PET/MR imaging index (ie, 0.933 vs 0.711, $P<.001$, respectively). The investigators concluded that the FDG-PET/MR imaging index yielded significantly improved specificity and diagnostic accuracy compared with conventional MR indices (MaRIA and the Clermont score).

FDG-PET/MR imaging has also been assessed for the evaluation of the aforementioned stenosis. In 2016, Catalano and colleagues[45] compared MR imaging, FDG-PET, and hybrid FDG-PET/MR imaging in terms of evaluating fibrotic strictures, using surgery as standard of reference. Combined FDG-PET/MR imaging was better than either examination alone. Best discriminator between fibrosis and active inflammation was the combined FDG-PET/MR-E apparent diffusion coefficient × SUV_{max} cutoff of less than 3000, which was associated with accuracy, sensitivity, and specificity values of 0.71, 0.67, and 0.73, respectively. Pellino and colleagues[46] showed FDG-PET/CT-E, FDG-PET/MR-E, and MR-E were equally accurate in detecting CD sites in a study enrolling 35 patients with known CD. PET/MR-E was found more accurate in detecting fibrotic components compared with FDG-PET/CT-E ($P = .043$) and with MR-E ($P = .024$). In conventional MR imaging, fibrosis was more frequently classified as inflammation compared with FDG-PET/MR-E ($P = .019$). After reviewing the FDG-PET-MR-E, 6 of 8 patients with predominantly inflammatory CD who received medical treatment remained surgery free (median follow-up of 9 [6–22] months).

DISCUSSION AND FUTURE PERSPECTIVE

Although FDG-PET/CT in IBD generally displays good sensitivity and specificity in different settings, many unanswered questions remain, and more evidence is needed. With continuous improvement of MR imaging and ultrasonography, these modalities continue to be the standard of care in most parts of the world. Internationally, a more widespread use of FDG-PET/CT as a universal, first-line modality for routine clinical practice is limited by availability, cost, and an appreciable radiation burden. The latter is especially important in IBD patients because most are diagnosed at a young age and often require repeated scans; the radiation reducing potential of PET/MR imaging and improved state-of-the-art PET/CT scanners are promising in this respect. Nonetheless, if FDG and PET/CT are to have a role in the future, they need to provide information not otherwise obtainable by MR imaging, ultrasound, or capsule endoscopy or as an adjunct in difficult cases.

The available literature points to several areas of potential, that is, early response evaluation especially in the setting of biologic treatment, assessment of strictures to guide treatment strategy, and diagnosis of extraintestinal disease. However, the literature is far from ideal; studies are generally small, with highly variable methodologies with regards to FDG-PET/CT, clinical parameters, treatment regimen, and reference standards. Thus, direct comparison or pooling of data is severely hampered. Add to this the intrinsic challenges of imaging the bowel, a moving organ with intrinsic physiologic activity and susceptibility to the effect of several extrinsic factors. Perhaps novel PET tracers with different or complementary properties could become a future game changer, but until now, none have been translated to human imaging.

With regards to reference standard, it is a striking feature of several studies that a significant proportion of included patients do not complete a full endoscopic examination (if such data are presented at all). A potential feature of FDG-PET/CT is the ability to detect disease proximal to endoscopy, but such lesions are often classified as false positives or excluded from data analysis even though they may represent true positive findings. Perhaps we also need to realize that a direct comparison between the morphologic and the functional modalities is far more difficult than usually appreciated with the dichotomous approach of most studies. Louis and colleagues[13] suggested that a large proportion of "false-positive" lesions on endoscopy may have contained subendoscopic features of activity on histology or involving deeper bowel layers. The suggestion from Louis et al. may be supported by a case report from Parbo and colleagues[47] on a young boy with UC on anti-TNF-α treatment who was clinically declining despite a normal colonoscopy. CT showed only discretely thickened walls of the colon, and small bowel capsule endoscopy showed no signs of inflammation. FDG-PET/CT scan was performed and revealed avid FDG uptake in the entire colon. An additional colonoscopy only indicated light disease activity, inconsistent with the clinical presentation. A total colectomy was performed, and subsequent pathologic examination of the colon showed multiple crypt abscesses under a healed mucosa. Similarly, in a study by Rubin and colleagues[48] FDG-PET/CT found inflammatory activity in the colon despite negative endoscopic, histology, and symptom assessment in 4 of 10 patients with known UC.

SUMMARY

To answer the question the authors posed in the title of this overview: Yes, the authors strongly believe there is a future role for FDG-PET/CT or FDG-PET/MR imaging in IBD. At present, most promising is the assessment of early treatment response and stricture characterization, whereas use in the initial diagnostic workup should be preserved for equivocal cases for the time being. However, there is a dire need for structured, well-designed prospective studies with strict protocols for patient preparation, imaging, and registration of clinical parameters and treatment regimens.

DISCLOSURE

The authors have nothing to disclose.

REFERENCES

1. Baumgart DC, Sandborn WJ. Crohn's disease. Lancet 2012;380(9853):1590–605.
2. Vind I, Riis L, Jess T, et al. Increasing incidences of inflammatory bowel disease and decreasing surgery rates in Copenhagen City and County, 2003-2005: a population-based study from the Danish Crohn colitis database. Am J Gastroenterol 2006;101(6):1274–82.
3. Binder V, Hendriksen C, Kreiner S. Prognosis in Crohn's disease–based on results from a regional patient group from the county of Copenhagen. Gut 1985;26(2):146–50.
4. Van Assche G, Dignass A, Panes J, et al. The second European evidence-based consensus on the diagnosis and management of Crohn's disease: definitions and diagnosis. J Crohns Colitis 2010;4:7–27.
5. Benitez JM, Meuwis MA, Reenaers C, et al. Role of endoscopy, cross-sectional imaging and biomarkers in Crohn's disease monitoring. Gut 2013;62(12):1806–16.
6. Kopylov U, Yung DE, Engel T, et al. Diagnostic yield of capsule endoscopy versus magnetic resonance enterography and small bowel contrast ultrasound in the evaluation of small bowel Crohn's disease: systematic review and meta-analysis. Dig Liver Dis 2017;49(8):854–63.
7. Jensen MD, Nathan T, Rafaelsen SR, et al. Diagnostic accuracy of capsule endoscopy for small bowel Crohn's disease is superior to that of MR enterography or CT enterography. Clin Gastroenterol Hepatol 2011;9(2):124–9.
8. Maaser C, Sturm A, Vavricka SR, et al. ECCO-ESGAR guideline for diagnostic assessment in IBD Part 1: initial diagnosis, monitoring of known IBD, detection of complications. J Crohns Colitis 2018;13(2):144–164K.
9. Toriihara A, Yoshida K, Umehara I, et al. Normal variants of bowel FDG uptake in dual-time-point PET/CT imaging. Ann Nucl Med 2011;25(3):173–8.
10. Tytgat GN. Hyoscine butylbromide–a review on its parenteral use in acute abdominal spasm and as an aid in abdominal diagnostic and therapeutic procedures. Curr Med Res Opin 2008;24(11):3159–73.
11. Emmott J, Sanghera B, Chambers J, et al. The effects of N-butylscopolamine on bowel uptake: an 18F-FDG PET study. Nucl Med Commun 2008;29(1):11–6.
12. Miraldi F, Vesselle H, Faulhaber PF, et al. Elimination of artifactual accumulation of FDG in PET imaging of colorectal cancer. Clin Nucl Med 1998;23(1):3–7.
13. Louis E, Ancion G, Colard A, et al. Noninvasive assessment of Crohn's disease intestinal lesions with (18)F-FDG PET/CT. J Nucl Med 2007;48(7):1053–9.
14. Koplay M, Guneyli S, Cebeci H, et al. Magnetic resonance enterography with oral mannitol solution: diagnostic efficacy and image quality in Crohn disease. Diagn Interv Imaging 2017;98(12):893–9.
15. Zhang L, Liang ML, Zhang YK, et al. The effects of hypotonic and isotonic negative contrast agent on gastrointestinal distention and physiological intake of 18F-FDG. Nucl Med Commun 2015;36(2):180–6.

16. Ozulker T, Ozulker F, Mert M, et al. Clearance of the high intestinal (18)F-FDG uptake associated with metformin after stopping the drug. Eur J Nucl Med Mol Imaging 2010;37(5):1011–7.

17. Hess S, Høilund-Carlsen PF, Alavi A. Historic images in nuclear medicine: 1976: the first issue of clinical nuclear medicine and the first human FDG study. Clin Nucl Med 2014 Aug;39(8):701–3. https://doi.org/10.1097/RLU.0000000000000487.

18. Hess S, Blomberg BA, Zhu HJ, et al. The pivotal role of FDG-PET/CT in modern medicine. Acad Radiol 2014;21(2):232–49.

19. Hess S, Alavi A, Basu S. PET-based personalized management of infectious and inflammatory disorders. PET Clin 2016;11(3):351–61.

20. Bicik I, Bauerfeind P, Breitbach T, et al. Inflammatory bowel disease activity measured by positron-emission tomography. Lancet 1997;350(9073):262.

21. Skehan SJ, Issenman R, Mernagh J, et al. F-18-fluorodeoxyglucose positron tomography in diagnosis of paediatric inflammatory bowel disease. Lancet 1999;354(9181):836–7.

22. Löffler M, Weckesser M, Franzius C, Schober O, Zimmer KP. High diagnostic value of 18F-FDG-PET in pediatric patients with chronic inflammatory bowel disease. Ann N Y Acad Sci. 2006 Aug;1072:379–85.

23. Das CJ, Makharia G, Kumar R, et al. PET-CT enteroclysis: a new technique for evaluation of inflammatory diseases of the intestine. Eur J Nucl Med Mol Imaging 2007;34(12):2106–14.

24. Neurath MF, Vehling D, Schunk K, et al. Noninvasive assessment of Crohn's disease activity: a comparison of F18-fluorodeoxyglucose positron emission tomography, hydromagnetic resonance imaging, and granulocyte scintigraphy with labeled antibodies. Am J Gastroenterol 2002;97(8):1978–85.

25. Lemberg DA, Issenman RM, Cawdron R, Green T, Mernagh J, Skehan SJ, Nahmias C, Jacobson K. Positron emission tomography in the investigation of pediatric inflammatory bowel disease. Inflamm Bowel Dis. 2005 Aug;11(8):733–8.

26. Meisner RS, Spier BJ, Einarsson S, et al. Pilot study using PET/CT as a novel, noninvasive assessment of disease activity in inflammatory bowel disease. Inflamm Bowel Dis 2007;13(8):993–1000.

27. Groshar D, Bernstine H, Stern D, et al. PET/CT enterography in Crohn disease: correlation of disease activity on CT enterography with F-18-FDG uptake. J Nucl Med 2010;51(7):1009–14.

28. Ahmadi A, Li Q, Muller K, et al. Diagnostic value of noninvasive combined Fluorine-18 labeled fluoro-2-deoxy-D-glucose positron emission tomography and computed tomography enterography in active Crohn's disease. Inflamm Bowel Dis 2010;16(6):974–81.

29. Shyn PB, Mortele KJ, Britz-Cunningham SH, et al. Low-dose 18F-FDG PET/CT enterography: improving on CT enterography assessment of patients with Crohn disease. J Nucl Med 2010;51(12):1841–8.

30. Das CJ, Makharia GK, Kumar R, et al. PET/CT colonography: a novel non-invasive technique for assessment of extent and activity of ulcerative colitis. Eur J Nucl Med Mol Imaging 2010;37(4):714–21.

31. Holtmann MH, Uenzen M, Helisch A, et al. 18F-Fluorodeoxyglucose positron-emission tomography (PET) can be used to assess inflammation non-invasively in Crohn's disease. Dig Dis Sci 2012;57(10):2658–68.

32. Treglia G, Quartuccio N, Sadeghi R, et al. Diagnostic performance of fluorine-18-fluorodeoxyglucose positron emission tomography in patients with chronic inflammatory bowel disease: a systematic review and a meta-analysis. J Crohns colitis 2013;7(5):345–54.

33. Jacene HA, Ginsburg P, Kwon J, et al. Prediction of the need for surgical intervention in obstructive Crohn's disease by F-18-FDG PET/CT. J Nucl Med 2009;50(11):1751–9.

34. Lenze F, Wessling J, Bremer J, et al. Detection and differentiation of inflammatory versus fibromatous Crohn's disease strictures: prospective comparison of 18F-FDG-PET/CT, MR-enteroclysis, and transabdominal ultrasound versus endoscopic/histologic evaluation. Inflamm Bowel Dis 2012;18(12):2252–60.

35. Spier BJ, Perlman SB, Jaskowiak CJ, et al. PET/CT in the evaluation of inflammatory bowel disease: studies in patients before and after treatment. Mol Imaging Biol 2010;12(1):85–8.

36. Russo EA, Khan S, Janisch R, et al. Role of 18F-fluorodeoxyglucose positron emission tomography in the monitoring of inflammatory activity in Crohn's disease. Inflamm Bowel Dis 2016;22(11):2619–29.

37. Epelboym Y, Shyn PB, Chick JFB, et al. Crohn disease: FDG PET/CT before and after initial dose of anti-tumor necrosis factor therapy to predict long-term response. Clin Nucl Med 2017;42(11):837–41.

38. Palatka K, Kacska S, Lovas S, et al. The potential role of FDG PET-CT in the characterization of the activity of Crohn's disease, staging follow-up and prognosis estimation: a pilot study. Scand J Gastroenterol 2018;53(1):24–30.

39. Hess S, Blomberg BA, Rakheja R, Friedman K, et al. A brief overview of novel approaches to FDG PET imaging and quantification. Clin Transl Imaging 2014;2:11.

40. Saboury B, Salavati A, Brothers A, et al. FDG PET/CT in Crohn's disease: correlation of quantitative FDG PET/CT parameters with clinical and endoscopic surrogate markers of disease activity. Eur J Nucl Med Mol Imaging 2014;41(4):605–14.

41. Berry N, Sinha SK, Bhattacharya A, et al. Role of positron emission tomography in assessing disease

activity in ulcerative colitis: comparison with bio-markers. Dig Dis Sci 2018;63(6):1541–50.

42. Domachevsky L, Leibovitzh H, Avni-Biron I, et al. Correlation of 18F-FDG PET/MRE metrics with inflammatory biomarkers in patients with Crohn's disease: a pilot study. Contrast Media Mol Imaging 2017;2017:7167292.

43. Li Y, Beiderwellen K, Nensa F, et al. [18F]FDG PET/MR enterography for the assessment of inflammatory activity in Crohn's disease: comparison of different MRI and PET parameters. Eur J Nucl Med Mol Imaging 2018;45(8):1382–93.

44. Li Y, Langhorst J, Koch AK, et al. Assessment of ileo-colonic inflammation in Crohn's disease: which surrogate marker is better-MaRIA, Clermont, or PET/MR index? Initial results of a feasibility trial. J Nucl Med 2019;60(6):851–7.

45. Catalano OA, Gee MS, Nicolai E, et al. Evaluation of quantitative PET/MR enterography biomarkers for discrimination of inflammatory strictures from fibrotic strictures in Crohn disease. Radiology 2016;278(3): 792–800.

46. Pellino G, Nicolai E, Catalano OA, et al. PET/MR versus PET/CT imaging: impact on the clinical management of small-bowel Crohn's disease. J Crohns Colitis 2016;10(3):277–85.

47. Parbo P, Stribolt K, Rittig CS, et al. Active ulcerative colitis diagnosed by (18)F-FDG PET/CT in an anti-TNF alpha treated patient with no visible luminal lesions on colonoscopy. Int J Colorectal Dis 2014; 29(5):643–4.

48. Rubin DT, Surma BL, Gavzy SJ, et al. Positron emission tomography (PET) used to image subclinical inflammation associated with ulcerative colitis (UC) in remission. Inflamm Bowel Dis 2009;15(5):750–5.

PET/Computed Tomography in Pulmonary and Thoracic Inflammatory Diseases (Including Cardiac Sarcoidosis)
The Current Role and Future Promises

Ashwini Kalshetty, DNB[a,b], Sandip Basu, DRM, DNB[a,b,*]

KEYWORDS

- Pulmonary inflammation • Thoracic inflammation • Sarcoidosis • COPD • FDG • PET/CT
- FLT-PET • ^{68}Ga-DOTANOC PET

KEY POINTS

- 18F-fluorodeoxyglucose PET/computed tomography (CT) can subserve as a valuable adjunct initial and posttreatment assessment of sarcoidosis, especially when conventional biomarkers and anatomic imaging are noncontributory and/or inconclusive.
- FDG-PET/CT is particularly useful in assessing therapeutic efficacy in sarcoidosis and can thereby influence clinical management.
- FDG-PET/CT can help in diagnosis and response assessment of cardiac sarcoidosis; however, new tracers could be helpful too without the requirement of tedious optimization and patient preparation protocols needed for cardiac FDG-PET/CT study. New tracers and technology could give major insights into the disease.
- Quantitative regional parameters of inflammation, perfusion, and ventilation estimated by PET/CT can help in the management of COPD by identifying and classifying into specific disease phenotypes.

INTRODUCTION

Restrictive and obstructive pulmonary diseases affect the general population globally. Thoracic inflammation is mostly diagnosed on anatomic imaging modalities, bronchoscopy, and histologic and microbiological evaluation. The spectrum of nonmalignant and noninfectious disease affecting lungs ranges from those affecting the interstitium to airspace and vasculature. The commonly encountered diseases include sarcoidosis and chronic obstructive pulmonary disease (COPD).

Aortoarteritis, Wegener granulomatous arteritis, systemic lupus erythematosus (SLE), and Kikuchi disease are other less common diseases, affecting the thorax as part of generalized inflammatory process. In systemic inflammatory disorders, ^{18}F-fluorodeoxyglucose (FDG)-PET/computed tomography (CT) functional molecular imaging serves 3 practical advantages compared with the conventional imaging modalities: (1) aiding in assessing entire body distribution of the disease in a single examination; (2) imaging the degree of inflammatory disease

[a] Radiation Medicine Centre (BARC), Tata Memorial Hospital Annexe, Parel, Mumbai 400012, India; [b] Homi Bhabha National Institute, Mumbai 400094, India
* Corresponding author. Radiation Medicine Centre, Bhabha Atomic Research Centre, Tata Memorial Hospital, Annexe Building, Jerbai Wadia Road, Parel, Mumbai 400 012, India.
E-mail address: drsanb@yahoo.com

PET Clin 15 (2020) 163–173
https://doi.org/10.1016/j.cpet.2019.11.008
1556-8598/20/© 2019 Elsevier Inc. All rights reserved.

activity; and (3) assessing the whole-body metabolic burden of inflammation, which is useful both at initial diagnosis and in posttherapeutic scenarios. This article describes the role of PET/CT in the diagnosis and management of inflammatory diseases in the lungs and thorax and explores its potential for precision medicine.

SARCOIDOSIS

Sarcoidosis is a systemic inflammatory disease of unknown cause, affecting most frequently the lungs; its etiopathogenesis has been elusive, with challenges in diagnosis and management, with pathognomonic noncaseating granulomas. The diagnosis of pulmonary sarcoidosis is established when the following 3 criteria are present: (1) compatible clinical and radiological diagnosis, (2) noncaseating granulomas on histopathology and (c) exclusion of other mimicking diseases.

The Scadding system of radiological classification is a simple tool based on chest radiography and divided into 5 stages (0– IV) and, although patients usually show disease progress from one stage to the next, the system always does not correlate well with disease severity, pulmonary function, and clinical decision making for tailoring treatment. High-resolution CT (HRCT) and serologic markers such as interleukin (IL)-2, angiotensin-converting enzyme (ACE) levels, and so forth provide complementary information for diagnosis of sarcoidosis, but they are of limited value in the management of patients. Bronchoscopy and bronchoscopy-guided biopsy are required for histologic confirmation. Around 20% to 30% of patients with pulmonary sarcoidosis may progress to pulmonary fibrosis and pulmonary hypertension, eventually leading to organ failure requiring transplant. The large-scale European multicenter GenPhenReSa (Genotype-Phenotype Relationship in Sarcoidosis) project was designed to study the influence of genotype on phenotype in sarcoidosis, based on multidimensional correspondence and cluster analysis. The results have shown 5 distinct organ-based phenotypes (according to predominant organ involvement): (1) abdominal, (2) ocular-cardiac-cutaneous–central nervous system, (3) musculoskeletal-cutaneous, (d4) pulmonary–lymph nodal, and (5) extrapulmonary.[1]

Investigators continue to search for a reliable biomarker that can reflect disease activity accurately, help in treatment monitoring, and provide information about other organ involvement by this systemic disease. FDG-PET/CT has the potential to give such information reliably. FDG has been shown to accumulate in the activated inflammatory cells of granulomas which correspond with the active site of inflammation. Visualizing and quantifying the metabolic activity on FDG-PET/CT gives information on the extent and severity of the disease and helps in disease management. **Fig. 1** shows the utility of FDG-PET/CT in initial evaluation of sarcoidosis.

TREATMENT RESPONSE MONITORING IN SARCOIDOSIS

It is been noticed often that serum ACE and IL-2 levels do not always correlate accurately with the disease activity during and after treatment.[2–5] Posttreatment FDG-PET/CT showing reduction in metabolic activity compared with the baseline suggests favorable treatment response, whereas persistence of metabolic activity suggests resistance to the administered therapy and may prompt the need to change the drugs. The newer quantitative parameters such as maximum standardized uptake value (SUVmax), mean standardized uptake value (SUVmean), metabolic index (maximum), and metabolic index (mean) are easily adoptable with the present generation of PET/CT scanners and provide objective complementary data, as shown in **Figs. 2** and **3**.

An area in which FDG-PET/CT has significant value is imaging documentation in patients with persistent symptoms suggesting steroid resistance.[2,3] **Fig. 3**A, B shows such a patient with persistent symptoms. The presence of steroid refractoriness has influenced clinical management by differentiating patients who may need tumor necrosis factor (TNF) alpha (infliximab) therapy earlier in the course of the disease.

The algorithm shown summarizes the established and the possible role of FDG-PET/CT in the management of sarcoidosis (**Fig. 4**). A possible future role of FDG-PET/CT that is also worth investigating is to identify high-risk pulmonary sarcoidosis that may have a potential role in disease phenotyping. However, these questions have not been addressed yet.

NON–[18]F-FLUORODEOXYGLUCOSE PET TRACERS IN SARCOIDOSIS

Non–FDG-PET tracers such as ^{68}Ga-DOTANOC[6,7] and [18]fluorothymidine (FLT)[8] have been studied for their potential role in imaging the disease activity, but further evidence is needed in this area. There is somatostatin receptor (SSTR) overexpression in sarcoid granulomas and, hence, SSTR imaging with ^{68}Ga-labeled somatostatin analogues could have a potential role in sarcoidosis. There is some preliminary evidence suggesting that SSTR expression suggests the acute phase of

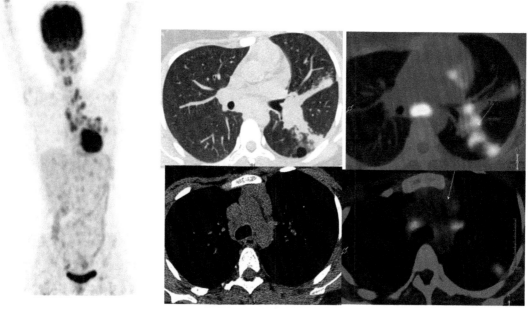

Fig. 1. A 22-year-old woman was initially suspected of pulmonary tuberculosis. However, on serial CT scans, there was progression of lung lesions with persistent thoracic nodes even following anti-tuberculosis drug (AKT). Serum angiotensin converting enzyme levels were marginally high at this point, 71 U/L with strong clinicoradiological suspicion of sarcoidosis. FDG-PET/CT showing hypermetabolic left lung lesions and thoracic nodes (including bilateral hilar nodes) (arrows). Low-grade uptake in thymus was also observed.

sarcoidosis.[6,7] SSTR imaging has the potential to identify granulomatous sites; however, poor contrast in areas of high background tracer uptake, such as in liver and spleen, may lead to low sensitivity and specificity.

CARDIAC SARCOIDOSIS

Cardiac sarcoidosis (CS) is commonly seen in patients around 25 to 45 years of age, with around a quarter of patients remaining asymptomatic. The remainder may present with typical features (conduction abnormalities, arrhythmias, heart failure) or sudden cardiac death. Between 20% and 25% of patients with systemic sarcoidosis are estimated to have cardiac involvement, whereas approximately 25% to 60% of patients have isolated CS.

The location and extent of involvement are associated with the clinical manifestations of CS.[9] There seems to be some predilection for the location of disease involvement to be the basal septum, left ventricular free wall, papillary muscles, and right ventricle, in descending order of frequency. The location and extent of cardiac involvement have been shown to have causal association with presenting symptoms. Pericardium may be involved too.

As per the recent guidelines, the potential role of cardiac FDG-PET/CT in the scenario of sarcoidosis is as follows[10]:

1. Known extracardiac sarcoidosis with suspected CS
2. Suspected CS
3. Response assessment in CS

The recent guidelines[9,10] have described the patient preparation protocols in detail. Meticulous preparation and optimization are required for the test and following them rigorously is not always convenient for the patient. The advantage with FDG-PET/CT is the whole-body screening for extracardiac involvement apart from regional PET/CT. As delineated by the guidelines,[10,11] interpretation requires both perfusion and metabolism images (**Table 1**). Visual as well as quantitative assessment is necessary for increasing sensitivity and accuracy of the study.

It has been noted that the focal-on-diffuse pattern (used as one of the interpretation criteria) when seen on FDG-PET/CT could be a physiologic variant and needs to be carefully distinguished from the pathologic uptake.[12]

QUANTITATIVE PET PARAMETERS FOR CARDIAC SARCOIDOSIS: REPORTED APPROACHES IN LITERATURE

In the study by Yokoyama and colleagues,[13] an SUVmax cutoff of greater than or equal to 4.0 had a sensitivity of 97.3% with a specificity of

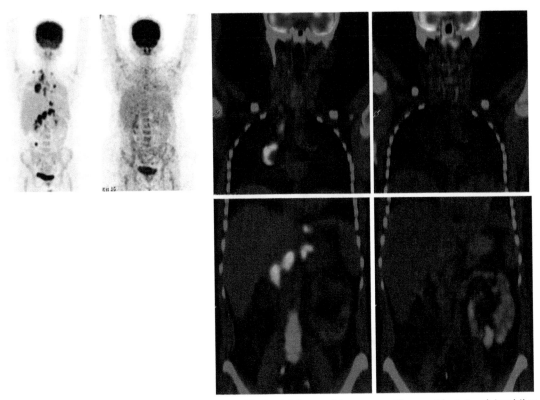

Fig. 2. FDG-PET/CT for treatment response in sarcoidosis. A 26-year-old woman with sarcoidosis involving bilateral lung, cervical, thoracic, and abdominal lymphadenopathy, treated with steroids. She had improvement of lung function after 3 months. FDG-PET/CT at 6 weeks (*right*; both maximum intensity projection [MIP] and fused coronal images) compared with baseline (*left*; both MIP and fused coronal images) shows complete metabolic resolution of lymphadenopathy. However, there was residual low-grade metabolic fibronodular changes in bilateral pulmonary parenchyma.

84.6% for the diagnosis of CS, with area under the curve by receiver operating characteristic analysis being 0.960 for the given SUVmax. Also, SUVmax decreased significantly in patients responsive to steroids.

In a study by Manabe and colleagues,[14] certain novel approaches have been proposed, such as (1) volume-based glucose metabolic analysis on FDG-PET/CT, with the boundary determined by a threshold (SUVmean of blood pool × 1.5), which could be of potential use as a promising parameter for diagnosing CS[13]; (b) uniformly adopting a fasting period longer than 18 hours to make the normal cardiac metabolic volume 0; and (c) adopting texture analysis and metabolic polar mapping.

PATIENT PREPARATION AND APPROACHES FOR CARDIAC SARCOIDOSIS IMAGING WITH ^{18}F-FLUORODEOXYGLUCOSE PET/ COMPUTED TOMOGRAPHY

The patient preparation and diet approaches for myocardial FDG-PET/CT imaging CS are

different. The fundamental principle and approaches for myocardial FDG-PET/CT imaging in CS are that, in inflammatory cells, glucose enters the cell via glucose transporter (GLUT) 1 and GLUT3 (overexpressed in tumors and inflammation), whereas glucose enters normal myocardial cells through the insulin-dependent GLUT4 GLUTs. Thus, active inflammation or granulomatous disease in myocardium by FDG-PET/CT imaging is better accomplished when there is a paucity or absence of carbohydrates and insulin (achieved by low carbohydrates and prolonged fasting), thereby shifting the myocardial metabolism toward free fatty acids for energy (further accentuated by high-fat, high-protein diet), which optimally suppresses physiologic myocardial uptake of FDG.

The popular approaches commonly used in clinical studies of CS imaging are (1) dietary (high fat, low/no carbohydrate), (2) short-term to long-term fasting, (3) coadministration of intravenous heparin 50 IU/kg (enhancing free fatty acids through pharmacologic lipolysis), and (4) calcium channel blockade with verapamil. The first 2 approaches

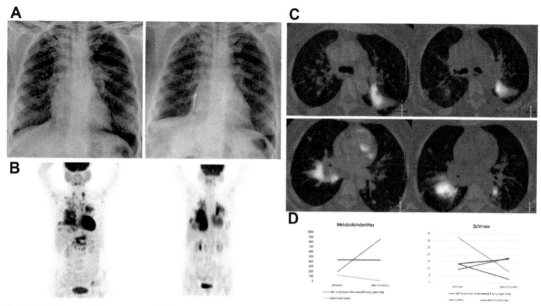

Fig. 3. A 55-year-old woman with known sarcoidosis having persistent dyspnea and cough even after treatment with steroids and methotrexate for 8 months. (*A*) Chest roentgenogram (CXR) showing reticulonodular changes seen in bilateral lung parenchyma with multiple interstitial nodules (right>left) in baseline CXR (*left upper*) along with right hilar prominence. Posttreatment CXR shows mild reduction of interstitial nodules and right hilar prominence. (*B*) Baseline PET/CT (*left*: MIP view) had shown metabolically active cervical and abdominal lymphadenopathy, bilateral pulmonary involvement, and diffuse cardiac uptake. Comparative FDG-PET MIP view at 8 months (*right*) shows persistence of FDG hypermetabolism in bilateral lungs and reduction of cardiac uptake and resolution of cervical and abdominal lymphadenopathy. (*C*) Comparative FDG-PET/CT (fused transaxial views) shows persistence of FDG hypermetabolism in pulmonary parenchyma. (*D*) Quantitative parameters showing increase in regional metabolic parameters in lungs. The quantitative parameters, SUVmax and metabolic index maximum showed increase in the pulmonary regions with decrease in cardiac uptake and cervical and abdominal lymphadenopathy.

are regularly used in clinical settings in most active PET centers.

NON–¹⁸F-FLUORODEOXYGLUCOSE PET TRACERS IN CARDIAC SARCOIDOSIS

In a study by Gormsen and colleagues,[12] ⁶⁸Ga-DOTANOC PET/CT had excellent diagnostic accuracy for diagnosing CS. In spite of prolonged fasting, a large proportion of FDG-PET/CT images were rated as inconclusive, and had poor diagnostic accuracy. By contrast, both interobserver agreement and accuracy were superior with ⁶⁸Ga-DOTANOC PET/CT, making this tracer more promising.[12]

A preliminary study by Norikane and colleagues[8] showed that FLT-PET/CT can detect cardiac and extracardiac thoracic involvement in patients with newly diagnosed sarcoidosis with a less inconclusive scan compared with FDG, although the cardiac uptake was lower compared with FDG. FLT was proposed to be a good alternative to FDG because it does not need special patient

preparation and there is no physiologic uptake in heart.

A comparison of tracers used in CS is given in **Table 2**.

Cardiac FDG-PET/CT may provide complementary information to cardiac magnetic resonance (MR) imaging, especially in inconclusive studies; may provide quantification of involvement; and may guide biopsy site and increase confidence of diagnosis.[15,16]

TREATMENT RESPONSE ASSESSMENT IN CARDIAC SARCOIDOSIS

FDG-PET/CT parameters are of potential use for assessing treatment response in CS. There is objective reduction of SUVmax and decrease in metabolic volume with successful therapy as well as improvement of left ventricular ejection fraction.[16]

DISEASE PROGNOSTICATION

The data are limited, but it is probable that patients with high FDG uptake and higher disease burden

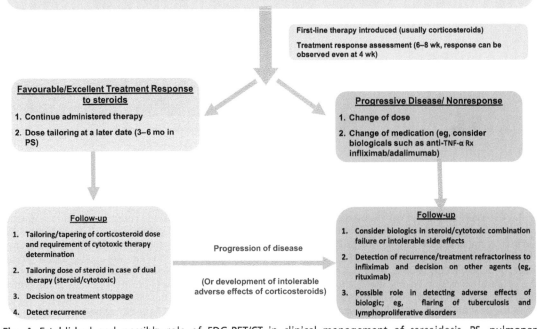

Fig. 4. Established and possible role of FDG-PET/CT in clinical management of sarcoidosis. PS, pulmonary sarcoidosis; Rx, therapy.

and probability of CS may show worse prognosis. Perfusion defects and abnormal metabolism on FDG-PET/CT predicted adverse events and were associated with death and ventricular tachycardia. The same group also reported that a focal uptake in the right ventricle was associated with poorer prognosis.[17]

CHRONIC OBSTRUCTIVE PULMONARY DISEASE

Globally, COPD is prevalent in roughly 3% of the population, with significant mortality and morbidity associated with it. Patients with COPD may present with progressive worsening of pulmonary function as well as frequent exacerbations and comorbidities leading to reduced quality of life and poor prognosis. The Global Initiative for Obstructive Lung Disease (GOLD) classification is currently used universally, and is robust with no absolute requisite of imaging. It considers clinical presentation and forced expiratory volume in 1 second (FEV1) values for classifying the disease. However, studies have highlighted the limitations of single FEV1 values, which have high interoperator and interpretation

variability.[18] This limitation is more profound in the management of mild to moderate cases of COPD. Volumetric/quantitative parameters on HRCT, dual-energy CT, and MR imaging have been evaluated and seem promising in objectively quantifying the disease load, but their impact on clinical management needs to be validated further. There are various other biomarkers for management, such as 6-minute walk distance, IL-6/IL-8, Clara cell protein (CC16), and C-reactive protein. However, all have their limitations the search for new biomarkers continues. Extensive research in COPD suggests that disease phenotyping could help in tailoring treatment and reducing morbidity.

FDG-PET/CT can have potential applications for disease phenotyping[19,20] (**Fig. 5**). Three clinically validated and commonly encountered phenotypes have been identified: (1) alpha-1 antitrypsin deficiency (AATD) related, (2) emphysema predominant, and (c) patients who get frequent exacerbations.

The current literature suggests FDG uptake in sites of neutrophilic inflammation in usual-type COPD.[20] This fundamental mechanism has been explored to distinguish the usual-type COPD (in

Table 1
Interpretation of ^{18}F-fluorodeoxyglucose PET–computed tomography in cardiac sarcoidosis

FDG Uptake	Perfusion Study	Probability (%)	Interpretation
—	Normal	<10	No CS
Nonspecific uptake	Small defect Normal	10–50	Possible CS
Focal Focal on diffuse Multiple areas of focal FDG uptake	Defect	50–90	Probable CS
Multiple areas of focal FDG uptake and extracardiac foci Multiple areas of focal FDG uptake	Multiple defects	>90	Highly probable

Data from Blankstein R, Waller AH. Evaluation of Known or Suspected Cardiac Sarcoidosis. Circ Cardiovasc Imaging. 2016 Mar;9(3):e000867 and Vita T, Okada DR, Veillet-Chowdhury M, Bravo PE, Mullins E, Hulten E, et al. Complementary Value of Cardiac Magnetic Resonance Imaging and Positron Emission Tomography/ Computed Tomography in the Assessment of Cardiac Sarcoidosis. Circ Cardiovasc Imaging. 2018 Jan;11(1):e007030.

which the etiopathogenesis is neutrophilic infiltration) from the AATD-type COPD.[20] This evidence also points toward a potential role of FDG-PET/CT in distinctly identifying the clinically encountered phenotypes and directing the treatment accordingly, as opposed to the anatomy-based quantitative parameters, which correlate weakly to such clinically relevant phenotypes.

A proposed model as per the recent literature is summarized in **Table 3**, which needs further examination in future studies.

Prospective clinical trials are needed to explore the clinical utility and validate the aforementioned proposition.

QUANTIFICATION OF INFLAMMATION

Various attempts have been made to quantify the inflammation in pulmonary parenchyma. However, the need to consider various factors, such as the various densities (airways, bronchioles, vasculature), motion correction, partial volume correction,

and a representative compartmental model, has led to tedious calculations and multiple parameters. The major techniques are summarized[21] in **Table 4**:

NEW AND NOVEL TRACERS TARGETING PULMONARY INFLAMMATION: RESULTS FROM IN VITRO AND ANIMAL STUDIES

Inducible nitric oxide synthase (NOS) is overexpressed in pulmonary inflammation. Preclinical and clinical studies have shown that ^{18}F-(+/ −)-NOS seems to specifically accumulate in areas of inflammation and could predict development of lung fibrosis.[22] Preclinical models have shown overexpression of chemokine receptor-2 (CCR2) in pulmonary inflammation.[23] There is an ongoing trial investigating biodistribution and dosimetry of Cu-DOTA-ECL1, which targets CCR2 expression in areas of active disease process. Another novel radiotracer is ^{18}F-fluciclatide, which is a radiolabeled polypeptide with affinity

Table 2
Comparison of tracers used in cardiac sarcoidosis

	FDG	FLT	^{68}Ga-DOTANOC
Patient Preparation	Meticulous preparation and prolonged fasting	Not required	Not required
Uptake	Increased in granulomas and reduced to absent in scar	Moderately increased in granulomas	Probably low (up to SUVmax 4)
Image Quality	Good	Low contrast	Low/interference by liver uptake
Usefulness Studied	For initial diagnosis and treatment response	Initial diagnosis	Proposed to be enhanced in acute phase

Data from Refs.[8,10,15]

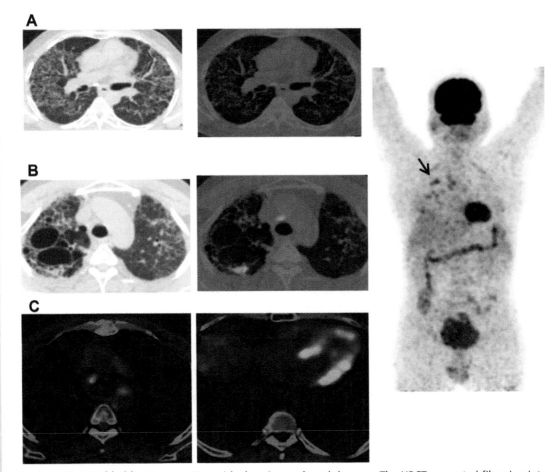

Fig. 5. A 50-year-old old man presenting with chronic cough and dyspnea. The HRCT suggested fibrosing interstitial lung disease. Transbronchial lung biopsy suggested bronchiectases with patchy interstitial fibrosis. FDG-PET/CT MIP image (*right*) shows patchy metabolic activity in bilateral lung fields (right>>left) and mediastinal nodes (*black arrows*). (*A*) Diffuse FDG uptake in bilateral ground-glass opacities, honeycombing, and interstitial septal nodularity. (*B*) Focal increased uptake in periphery of bronchiectatic changes seen in right lung upper lobe, suggesting ongoing inflammatory disease process likely to show progression. (*C*) Metabolically active mediastinal nodes.

for αvβ3/αvβ5 integrin and is a potential marker for angiogenesis and activated fibroblasts.[22] These new radiotracers open a new avenue of in vivo mapping of disease pathogenesis, and accurate representation of areas of inflammation along with fibrosis may be possible. These radiotracers could also lead to new drug development and testing.

QUANTIFICATION OF REGIONAL VENTILATION/PERFUSION WITH PET

A few studies that explored regional ventilation/perfusion with non–FDG-PET tracers are enumerated here:

1. [13]N was used to map regional ventilation and perfusion by Vidal Melo and colleagues.[24] The study showed that there is more heterogeneous regional perfusion in patients with COPD than in healthy people. There was also loss of a regional ventilation gradient, and heterogeneity of ventilation-perfusion ratios was also larger in subjects with COPD compared with healthy subjects.

2. ^{68}Ga-labeled carbon nanoparticles and ^{68}Ga-Macroaggregated albumin (MAA) have also been used to delineate high-resolution functional regional ventilation and perfusion areas.[25] The volumetric fraction of perfusion and ventilation greater than or equal to 90% was shown to identify COPD cases with a sensitivity of 93%.[26,27] Four-dimensional gated acquisitions might increase the accuracy of delineating functional volumes.[25]

Table 3
Correlation of ^{18}F-fluorodeoxyglucose uptake with clinical phenotypes of chronic obstructive pulmonary disease

	AATD-Related COPD	Emphysema-Predominant COPD	COPD with Frequent Exacerbations
Treatment	Augmentation therapy	Reduction surgery	Hospitalization and supportive treatment
FDG Uptake	Low	Mild to moderate	Moderate to high (theoretically)

Data from Subramanian DR, Jenkins L, Edgar R, Quraishi N, Stockley RA, Parr DG. Assessment of pulmonary neutrophilic inflammation in emphysema by quantitative positron emission tomography. Am J Respir Crit Care Med. 2012 Dec 1;18(11):1125-32.

INDIRECT BIOMARKERS OF SEVERITY: CORRELATION WITH PULMONARY FUNCTION TESTS

There are several indirect markers for severity of disease to be recognized on FDG-PET/CT images[28–31]:

1. Decrease in FDG metabolism over time in the left ventricle corresponds with the severity of obstruction and could be associated with right ventricle overload and pulmonary arterial hypertension.
2. Increase of the right ventricular metabolism could be a substitute marker for severity of COPD and smoking.
3. Increased uptake in respiratory muscles suggests presence of COPD, predominantly in intercostal muscles.

PROGNOSTICATION OF CHRONIC OBSTRUCTIVE PULMONARY DISEASE AND INTERSTITIAL LUNG DISEASE

FDG-PET/CT has been investigated for its potential for monitoring and risk stratification of patients with interstitial lung disease (ILD). In a study by Nobashi and colleagues[32] in 90 patients with ILD (compared with 15 age-matched and sex-matched healthy controls), SUVmean of the affected lung field, SUV_{mean} using tissue fraction, and mean attenuation of the corresponding region of interest on HRCT (CT_{mean}) were significantly higher in patients with ILD than in healthy controls. The investigators concluded that SUV_{mean} was significantly correlated with clinical indicators, providing independent prognostic information in patients with ILD. Higher SUV_{mean} suggested a poorer prognosis.

SYSTEMIC LUPUS ERYTHEMATOSUS

Akin to other systemic inflammatory disorders, FDG-PET/CT could aid in the management of SLE in the following ways: (1) assessing whole-body distribution of the disease, (2) improving the ability to visualize the degree of disease activity, and (3) assessing the whole-body metabolic burden of inflammation. In untreated patients, FDG-PET/CT shows widespread lymphadenopathy and increased thymic uptake in SLE. The

Table 4
Major techniques in quantification of ^{18}F-fluorodeoxyglucose

Quantitative FDG-PET Parameters	Measures	Advantage	Disadvantage
Semiquantitative SUV	Activity concentration per body weight corrected to time	Simple	Variable and prone to errors
Graphical analysis Patlak analysis	Net pulmonary uptake rate (Ki)	Effective	Limited because dynamic TAC needed
Compartmental analysis Kinetic modeling	Net pulmonary uptake rate (Ki)	Theoretically more accurate if lung-specific model is developed	Accurate modeling needs to be devised Technically demanding

Abbreviation: TAC, time activity curve.

uptake is indistinguishable from active lymphoma or tuberculosis, but FDG-PET/CT–guided biopsy may help in characterization of the lesions.[33–35]

Myocarditis is known to be associated with SLE (known as lupus myocarditis [LM]), which is considered to be the cause of congestive heart failure (CHF), one of the leading causes of death in patients with SLE. Perel-Winkler and colleagues[36] studied 8 patients with presumed LM and reported diffuse uptake in myocardium in 50% of the patients (who also had a decreased ejection fraction on echocardiography), suggesting myocardial inflammation. The patients were treated with high-dose steroids based on the diagnosis of LM. Further studies need to be undertaken, including its possible role in treatment response monitoring in LM.

SUMMARY

PET/CT imaging with FDG and other non-FDG tracers has shown potential to provide insights into pathogenesis, phenotyping, and staging of disease in pulmonary and thoracic inflammatory disorders. The major strengths are objective documentation and assessment of disease activity, and early treatment response evaluation, whereby it can influence clinical management in several disorders, such as sarcoidosis, whereas for COPD and ILDs it shows potential for disease risk stratification.[37–39] Its use may help in further refining the present understanding of these inflammatory disorders and paving the way for new drug development.

REFERENCES

1. Schupp JC, Freitag-Wolf S, Bargagli E, et al. Phenotypes of organ involvement in sarcoidosis. Eur Respir J 2018;51(1) [pii:1700991].
2. Keijsers RG, van den Heuvel DA, Grutters JC. Imaging the inflammatory activity of sarcoidosis. Eur Respir J 2013;41(3):743–51.
3. Sobic-Saranovic D, Artiko V, Obradovic V. FDG PET imaging in sarcoidosis. Semin Nucl Med 2013;43(6):404–11.
4. Ambrosini V, Zompatori M, Fasano L, et al. (18)F-FDG PET/CT for the assessment of disease extension and activity in patients with sarcoidosis: results of a preliminary prospective study. Clin Nucl Med 2013;38(4):e171–7.
5. Treglia G, Annunziata S, Sobic-Saranovic D, et al. The role of 18F-FDG-PET and PET/CT in patients with sarcoidosis: an updated evidence-based review. Acad Radiol 2014;21(5):675–84.
6. Slart RHJA, Koopmans KP, van Geel PP, et al. Somatostatin receptor based hybrid imaging in sarcoidosis. Eur J Hybrid Imaging 2017;1(1):7.
7. Nobashi T, Nakamoto Y, Kubo T, et al. The utility of PET/CT with (68)Ga-DOTATOC in sarcoidosis: comparison with (67)Ga-scintigraphy. Ann Nucl Med 2016;30(8):544–52.
8. Norikane T, Yamamoto Y, Maeda Y, et al. Comparative evaluation of (18)F-FLT and (18)F-FDG for detecting cardiac and extra-cardiac thoracic involvement in patients with newly diagnosed sarcoidosis. EJNMMI Res 2017;7(1):69.
9. Birnie DH, Nery PB, Ha AC, et al. Cardiac sarcoidosis. J Am Coll Cardiol 2016;68(4):411–21.
10. Chareonthaitawee P, Beanlands RS, Chen W, et al. Joint SNMMI-ASNC expert consensus document on the role of (18)F-FDG PET/CT in cardiac sarcoid detection and therapy monitoring. J Nucl Cardiol 2017;24(5):1741–58.
11. Writing group, Document reading group, EACVI Reviewers, This document was reviewed by members of the EACVI Scientific Documents Committee for 2014–2016 and 2016–2018. A joint procedural position statement on imaging in cardiac sarcoidosis: from the cardiovascular and inflammation & infection Committees of the European Association of Nuclear Medicine, the European Association of Cardiovascular Imaging, and the American Society of Nuclear Cardiology. Eur Heart J Cardiovasc Imaging 2017;18(10):1073–89.
12. Gormsen LC, Haraldsen A, Kramer S, et al. A dual tracer (68)Ga-DOTANOC PET/CT and (18)F-FDG PET/CT pilot study for detection of cardiac sarcoidosis. EJNMMI Res 2016;6(1):52.
13. Yokoyama R, Miyagawa M, Okayama H, et al. Quantitative analysis of myocardial 18F-fluorodeoxyglucose uptake by PET/CT for detection of cardiac sarcoidosis. Int J Cardiol 2015;195:180–7.
14. Manabe O, Kroenke M, Aikawa T, et al. Volume-based glucose metabolic analysis of FDG PET/CT: the optimum threshold and conditions to suppress physiological myocardial uptake. J Nucl Cardiol 2019;26(3):909–18.
15. Vita T, Okada DR, Veillet-Chowdhury M, et al. Complementary value of cardiac magnetic resonance imaging and positron emission tomography/computed tomography in the assessment of cardiac sarcoidosis. Circ Cardiovasc Imaging 2018;11(1):e007030.
16. Bravo PE, Singh A, Di Carli MF, et al. Advanced cardiovascular imaging for the evaluation of cardiac sarcoidosis. J Nucl Cardiol 2019;26(1):188–99.
17. Blankstein R, Osborne M, Naya M, et al. Cardiac positron emission tomography enhances prognostic assessments of patients with suspected cardiac sarcoidosis. J Am Coll Cardiol 2014;63(4):329–36.

18. Schermer TR, Robberts B, Crockett AJ, et al. Should the diagnosis of COPD be based on a single spirometry test? NPJ Prim Care Respir Med 2016;26: 16059.

19. Lange P, Halpin DM, O'Donnell DE, et al. Diagnosis, assessment, and phenotyping of COPD: beyond FEV1. Int J Chron Obstruct Pulmon Dis 2016;11 Spec Iss:3–12.

20. Subramanian DR, Jenkins L, Edgar R, et al. Assessment of pulmonary neutrophilic inflammation in emphysema by quantitative positron emission tomography. Am J Respir Crit Care Med 2012; 18(11):1125–32.

21. Schroeder T, Melo MF, Venegas JG. Analysis of 2-[Fluorine-18]-Fluoro-2-deoxy-D-glucose uptake kinetics in PET studies of pulmonary inflammation. Acad Radiol 2011;18(4):418–23.

22. Chen DL, Schiebler ML, Goo JM, et al. PET imaging approaches for inflammatory lung diseases: current concepts and future directions. Eur J Radiol 2017; 86:371–6.

23. Liu Y, Gunsten SP, Sultan DH, et al. PET-based imaging of chemokine receptor 2 in experimental and disease-related lung inflammation. Radiology 2017; 283(3):758–68.

24. Vidal Melo MF, Winkler T, Harris RS, et al. Spatial heterogeneity of lung perfusion assessed with (13)N PET as a vascular biomarker in chronic obstructive pulmonary disease. J Nucl Med 2010;51(1):57–65.

25. Callahan J, Hofman MS, Siva S, et al. High-resolution imaging of pulmonary ventilation and perfusion with 68Ga-VQ respiratory gated (4-D) PET/CT. Eur J Nucl Med Mol Imaging 2014;41(2):343–9.

26. Le Roux PY, Hicks RJ, Siva S, et al. PET/CT lung ventilation and perfusion scanning using galligas and gallium-68-MAA. Semin Nucl Med 2019;49(1): 71–81.

27. Jahangiri P, Pournazari K, Khosravi M, et al. Assessment of the correlation between pulmonary parenchymal inflammation and pulmonary function test indices in COPD patients using partial volume corrected FDG-PET/CT parameters. J Nucl Med 2018; 59(supplement 1):518.

28. Choi GG, Han Y, Weston B, et al. Metabolic effects of pulmonary obstruction on myocardial functioning: a pilot study using multiple time-point 18F-FDG-PET imaging. Nucl Med Commun 2015;36(1):78–83.

29. von Siebenthal C, Aubert JD, Mitsakis P, et al. Pulmonary hypertension and indicators of right ventricular function. Front Med (Lausanne) 2016;3:23.

30. Osman MM, Tran IT, Muzaffar R, et al. Does 18F-FDG uptake by respiratory muscles on PET/CT correlate with chronic obstructive pulmonary disease? J Nucl Med Technol 2011;39(4):252–7.

31. Basu S, Alzeair S, Li G, et al. Etiopathologies associated with intercostal muscle hypermetabolism and prominent right ventricle visualization on 2-deoxy-2[F-18]fluoro-D-glucose-positron emission tomography: significance of an incidental finding and in the setting of a known pulmonary disease. Mol Imaging Biol 2007;9(6):333–9.

32. Nobashi T, Kubo T, Nakamoto Y, et al. 18F-FDG uptake in less affected lung field provides prognostic stratification in patients with interstitial lung disease. J Nucl Med 2016;57(12):1899–904.

33. Curiel R, Akin EA, Beaulieu G, et al. PET/CT imaging in systemic lupus erythematosus. Ann N Y Acad Sci 2011;1228:71–80.

34. Kong E, Chun K, Hong Y, et al. 18F-FDG PET/CT findings in patients with Kikuchi disease. Nuklearmedizin 2013;52(3):101–6.

35. Zhang X, Xu C, Wang X. (18)F-FDG PET/CT imaging in systemic lupus erythematosus related autoimmune haemolytic anaemia and lymphadenopathy. Hell J Nucl Med 2016;19(1):42–5.

36. Perel-Winkler A, Bokhari S, Perez-Recio T, et al. Myocarditis in systemic lupus erythematosus diagnosed by (18)F-fluorodeoxyglucose positron emission tomography. Lupus Sci Med 2018;5(1): e000265.

37. Basu S, Saboury B, Werner T, et al. Clinical utility of FDG-PET and PET/CT in non-malignant thoracic disorders. Mol Imaging Biol 2011;13(6):1051–60.

38. Basu S, Yadav M, Joshi J. Potential of 18F-FDG-PET and PET/CT in nonmalignant pulmonary disorders: much more than currently perceived? Making the case from experience gained in the Indian scenario. Nucl Med Commun 2014;35(7):689–96.

39. Yadav M, Karkhanis VS, Basu S, et al. Potential clinical utility of FDG-PET in non-malignant pulmonary disorders: a pilot study. Indian J Chest Dis Allied Sci 2016;58(3):165–72.

FDG-PET/CT in Fever of Unknown Origin, Bacteremia, and Febrile Neutropenia

Søren Hess, MD[a,b],*

KEYWORDS

- FDG • PET • PET/CT • Fever of unknown origin • Bacteremia • Febrile neutropenia • Infection

KEY POINTS

- The literature on fever of unknown origin (FUO), bacteremia, and febrile neutropenia is generally heterogeneous and mainly based on small retrospective series; in bacteremia and febrile neutropenia series are few.
- FUO, bacteremia, and febrile neutropenia are diagnostic challenges; FDG-PET/CT is a well-established modality and should be considered early in the diagnostic work-up algorithm.
- In FUO, FDG-PET/CT is overall helpful in half the patients even after extensive work-up and superior to gamma camera–based radionuclide modalities, but diagnostic yield is highly dependent on patient selection (eg, clear definition of FUO), and a mandatory presence of elevated inflammatory markers (eg, C-reactive protein).
- FDG-PET/CT is cost-effective in establishing metastatic infection in bacteremia with impact on morbidity, mortality, and treatment strategy.

INTRODUCTION

Fever of unknown origin (FUO), bacteremia, and febrile neutropenia share some common features, such as heterogeneous patient populations and potential systemic nature, but often vague or nonspecific symptoms unable to locate the origin of disease. Imaging is pivotal to establish a final diagnosis, but despite the availability of multiple modalities, a significant proportion of patients remain underdiagnosed. FDG-PET/CT has potential in all three domains, but at present no definitive diagnostic strategy is established in either setting. This review summarizes the current evidence for the use of FDG-PET/CT with a focus on potential, challenges and caveats.

FEVER OF UNKNOWN ORIGIN

FUO remains a challenging clinical entity; patient populations are heterogeneous, and diagnostic clues are often sparse, nonspecific, or nonexisting. Although final diagnosis may overall be categorized as infection, noninfectious inflammatory disease, malignancy, or miscellaneous, more than 200 specific differential diagnoses are recognized,[1] and despite extensive diagnostic work-up a firm final diagnosis is never reached in a significant proportion of patients. In the papers included here the fraction of patients without a final diagnosis ranged from 0% to 47% (**Table 1**). Since the first definition by Petersdorf and Beeson[2] in 1961, modifications have been implemented to reflect a health care

[a] Department of Radiology and Nuclear Medicine, Hospital of Southwest Jutland, Finsensgade 35, Esbjerg 6700, Denmark; [b] Department of Regional Health Research, University of Southern Denmark, Odense, Denmark
* Department of Radiology and Nuclear Medicine, Hospital of Southwest Jutland, Finsensgade 35, Esbjerg 6700, Denmark.
E-mail address: soeren.hess@rsyd.dk

PET Clin 15 (2020) 175–185
https://doi.org/10.1016/j.cpet.2019.11.002
1556-8598/20/© 2019 Elsevier Inc. All rights reserved.

system increasingly based on out-patient activity (**Table 2**).[1]

In the past two decades, radionuclide imaging in FUO has shifted more and more from classic gamma camera–based imaging toward FDG-PET and FDG-PET/CT. This is supported not only by the increasing availability of PET/CT scanners, better logistics with faster results, and avoidance of handling patient blood, but also several comparative studies with results that generally favored FDG-PET or FDG-PET/CT over [67]gallium-citrate (^{67}Ga-citrate) or labeled white blood cells (WBC). An early prospective comparison of FDG-PET and the then gold standard whole-body planar ^{67}Ga-citrate in 58 patients yielded a final diagnosis in 64%; FDG-PET was helpful in 35%, ^{67}Ga-citrate in 25%, and all ^{67}Ga-positive findings were also FDG-avid. Thus, the authors concluded (based on better logistics and noninferior results) that FDG-PET could replace ^{67}Ga-citrate.[3] A recent study prospectively compared FDG-PET/CT with ^{67}Ga-citrate single-photon emission CT/CT in 58 patients and found the two helpful in 72% and 55%, respectively, with a false-positive rate of 44% in FDG-PET/CT and a false-negative rate of 55% with ^{67}Ga-citrate.[4]

An early prospective comparison of [111]indium-labelled WBC scintigraphy (^{111}In-WBC) and FDG-PET/CT at first glance strongly favored ^{111}In-WBC, that is, sensitivity and specificity was

---

Table 1
Selected papers on diagnostic efficacy of FDG-PET/CT in fever of unknown origin

Author (year)	Modality	N	Design	Final Diagnosis	Helpful (Essential)
Lorenzen et al,[9] 2001	PET	16	Prospective	N.R.	69%[a]
Bleeker-Rovers et al,[10] 2004	PET	35	Retrospective	54%	37%
Buysschaert et al,[11] 2004	PET	110	Prospective	53%	26%
Jaruskova and Belohlavek,[12] 2006	Mixed	118	Retrospective	N.R.	36%
Bleeker-Rovers et al,[13] 2007	PET	70	Prospective	50%	33%[a]
Vanderschueren et al,[14] 2009	PET	90	Prospective	58%	36%[a]
Kubota et al,[15] 2011	Mixed	81	Retrospective	67%	51%[a] 73%[b]
Keidar et al,[16] 2008	PET/CT	48	Retrospective	60%	46%[a]
Balink et al,[17] 2009	PET/CT	68	Retrospective	65%	56%[a]
Federici et al,[18] 2010	PET/CT	14	Retrospective	71%	50% (23%)
Ferda et al,[19] 2010	PET/CT	48	Retrospective	100%	92%
Kei et al,[20] 2010	PET/CT	12	Retrospective	58%	42%
Rosenbaum et al,[21] 2011	PET/CT	18	Retrospective	100%	N.R.
Sheng et al,[22] 2011	PET/CT	48	Retrospective	75%	N.R.
Pelosi et al,[23] 2011	PET/CT	24	Retrospective	71%	46%[a]
Ergül et al, 2011	PET/CT	24	Retrospective	79%	50%[a]
Crouzet et al,[25] 2012	PET/CT	79	Retrospective	77%	57%
Kim et al,[26] 2012	PET/CT	48	Retrospective	85%	66%[b]
Pedersen et al,[27] 2012	PET/CT	52	Retrospective	60%	45%
Manohar et al,[28] 2013	PET/CT	103	Retrospective	67%	61%[a]
Tokmak et al,[29] 2014	PET/CT	25	Retrospective	92%	60%[a]
Buch-Olsen et al,[30] 2014	PET/CT	57	Retrospective	86%	75%[b]
Gafter-Gvili et al,[31] 2015	PET/CT	112	Retrospective	74%	66%[b]
Singh et al,[35] 2015	PET/CT	47	Retrospective	54%	38% (6%)
Bouter et al,[32] 2016	PET/CT	72	Retrospective	83%	65% (40%)[a]
Schönau et al,[75] 2018	PET/CT	240	Prospective	79%	57%
Abdelrahman et al,[34] 2018	PET/CT	27	Prospective	93%	85[a]
Wang et al,[36] 2019	PET/CT	376	Retrospective	91%	77%

Abbreviation: N.R., not reported.
  [a] Only FDG-positive (true-positive) findings were considered helpful.
  [b] Both FDG-positive and FDG-negatives (true-positive and true-negative) findings were considered helpful.

Table 2
Original and current definitions of fever of unknown origin (based on[1])

Original Definition by Petersdorf et al,[2] 1961	Current Definition
Temperature >38.3°C (101°F) on 3 or more occasions	Temperature >38.3°C (101°F) on 2 or more occasions
Duration of illness >3 weeks	Duration of illness >3 weeks
No diagnosis after 1 wk admission (later revised to 3 days admission or 3 out-patient visits)	Not immunocompromised No definitive diagnosis despite thorough history-taking; physical examination; and a series of predefined initial investigations including a multitude of inflammatory markers and basic serology, urinalysis, blood cultures, urine culture, chest radiograph, abdominal ultrasound, and tuberculin skin test

71% and 92% versus 50% and 46%, respectively, but some caveats of potential selection and verification bias pertain to this study.[5,6] Thus, a later prospective study of 23 patients yielded opposite results, that is, sensitivity and specificity of 86% and 78% (FDG-PET/CT) versus 20% and 100% (^{111}In-WBC).[7]

A recent meta-analysis strongly favors FDG-PET/CT with sensitivities/specificities for FDG-PET/CT, FDG-PET, ^{67}Ga-citrate, and WBC scintigraphy of 86%/52%, 76%/50%, 60%/63%, and 33%/83%, respectively, and an overall diagnostic yield in the four modalities of 58%, 44%, 35%, and 20%, respectively.[8]

The studies with a focus on diagnostic accuracy of FDG-PET and FDG-PET/CT in FUO (see **Table 1**) comprise the bulk of the available literature,[9–36] although the list is not considered exhaustive because the literature search was not systematic. They also reflect the heterogeneous nature of the populations and methodologies, including variable reference standards, and the challenges related to this particular setting; definitions of FUO vary considerably (some also include inflammation of unknown origin [IUO], that is, prolonged elevation of inflammatory markers without fever), which hampers direct comparison of study populations; most use FDG-PET/CT, although a few of the older papers are based on stand-alone PET; and only a few series are prospective. Populations are generally small (median, 48 patients; range, 12–376), and a final diagnosis is not reached in all patients (median, 71%; range, 50%–100%).

How to assess the diagnostic value of FDG-PET/CT in the setting of FUO is controversial. Instead of classic diagnostic parameters, such as sensitivity and specificity, which may be difficult to define and dichotomize with the abundance of potential differential diagnosis, most studies report the proportion of patients in whom FDG-PET/CT was considered helpful in the diagnostic process (median, 54%; range, 26%–92%). However, how helpful is defined is also a matter of debate (eg, only true-positive findings that provide direct guidance to the clinician by establishing a diagnosis directly based on FDG-uptake; or if also true-negative findings that may rule out focal infection, inflammation, or malignancies with a high negative predictive value [NPV] and generally holds favorable prognosis). For instance, Pelosi and colleagues[23] defined only true-positives as helpful, that is, 46% (11 FDG-positive patients of 24), but if the 10 true-negatives were also considered helpful the rate would increase to 88%. Jaruskova and Belohlavek[12] directly characterized 67 negative FDG-PET/CT scans as not helpful. Conversely, for example, Keidar and colleagues[16] also considered true-negatives as helpful and reported an NPV of 100%, and Bleeker-Rovers and colleagues[37] categorized 34 FDG-negative scans as true-negative.

Another highly variable issue is the diagnostic pathways before FDG-PET/CT, which may contribute significantly to heterogeneity and potentially introduce selection bias. Some studies present comparative data on FDG-PET or FDG-PET/CT versus CT, such as Manohar and colleagues[28] with sensitivity, specificity, and accuracy of FDG-PET/CT being 90%, 97%, and 92%, respectively, versus 44%, 67%, and 52%, respectively, for CT. Bleeker-Rovers and colleagues[37] found positive predictive value (PPV) and NPV for FDG-PET (65% and 90%) better than for CT (48% and 86%), whereas Rosenbaum and colleagues[21] found 100% PPV for FDG-PET compared with 39% for diagnostic CT.

Most studies use several diagnostic modalities before referral to FDG-PET/CT. For example, Buch-Olsen and colleagues[30] reported that 57 patients underwent 126 examinations before FDG-PET/CT (not including chest radiograph and ultrasound of the abdomen, which comprised the local initial routine work-up in FUO). The earlier FDG-PET/CT is introduced the higher the potential impact because every imaging modality performed before FDG-PET/CT may potentially make a diagnosis and select patients to not undergo further modalities, thus leaving the harder cases to FDG-PET/CT. For instance, Ferda and colleagues[19] reported the highest rate of helpfulness (92%), and they used FDG-PET/CT as entry method to the study.

Only limited data are available on cost-effectiveness, but according to Buch-Olsen and colleagues[30] basic cost of FDG-PET/CT was covered if admission time was shortened by only 2.2 days, which is not unrealistic when considering the potential for precisely guided therapy.

The relative abundance of studies on FUO is reflected in several systematic reviews and meta-analysis available. However, the previously mentioned caveats and differences among studies are also reflected in the heterogeneity that is present in all of them including the variable outcome measures in the various papers. The two oldest[38,39] and the newest[40] all focused on pooled sensitivity and specificity, that is, 83% to 98% and 58% to 86%, respectively, with a tendency toward better sensitivity and specificity with FDG-PET/CT than stand-alone FDG-PET. It is worth mentioning that Hao and colleagues[39] included and pooled values from several different settings of FUO including human immunodeficiency virus, intensive care unit patients, and pediatric populations, whereas Kan and colleagues[40] pooled both FUO and IUO. Besson and colleagues[41] found that abnormal FDG uptake was associated with a final diagnosis in 83% versus only 36% in patients with a normal FDG-PET/CT, whereas Bharucha and colleagues[42] found an overall diagnostic yield of 56%, which was reduced to 32% in patients who had undergone diagnostic CT before FDG-PET/CT. Finally, Takeuchi and colleagues[43] found that patients had a high likelihood of spontaneous remission with a normal FDG-PET/CT after a series of diagnostic procedures without final diagnosis.

FDG-PET/CT has also been explored in more specialized cases of FUO (eg, human immunodeficiency virus). Two small series, one retrospective (n = 10) and one prospective (n = 20), found FDG-PET/CT helpful in 80% to 90% of patients,[44,45] and the prospective study found FDG-uptake in central lymph nodes to be associated with focal infection with 100% specificity, whereas absence of FDG in central lymph nodes had 100% NPV with regards to focal infection.[45] Also in critically ill intensive care unit patients has FDG-PET/CT shown potential, that is, sensitivity and specificity of 100% and 79%, respectively. The study included 33 patients with 17 being investigated for FUO, and in line with the conventional FUO patients mentioned previously most patients had undergone extensive work-up before FDG-PET/CT (eg, either echocardiography or CT in two-thirds of the patients).[46]

Studies in various pediatric settings have found similar results. Two retrospective studies examined children with FUO in 69[47] and 31 patients,[48] respectively. Final diagnosis was reached in 54% and 52%, respectively, and FDG PET or FDG-PET/CT was considered helpful in 32% and 45%, respectively.[47,48] Sturm and colleagues[49] examined 11 children with FUO while waiting for liver transplantation; five were positive with intrahepatic FDG-uptake and based on these findings the patients underwent transplantation after continuous antibiotic treatment and images correlated with bacterial cultures from the excised livers in all patients.

To optimize the usage of FDG-PET/CT in FUO several of the previously mentioned diagnostic studies have included some assessments of factors that may influence or predict the diagnostic yield, such as adenopathy and low hemoglobin levels,[25] short disease course,[31] and age greater than 50 years,[33] whereas others did not find inflammatory markers to predict positive findings.[11] A few studies have focused more directly on potential predictors of diagnostic success, and suspected malignancies, the number of positive inflammatory markers, and increasing values of C-reactive protein (CRP) and erythrocyte sedimentation rate all seemed positively correlated with positive yield or greater likelihood of a beneficial result.[50–52] Overall, no firm conclusions or cut-offs are established, but one study found FDG-PET/CT 100% negative in patients with CRP values less than 5 mg/L,[50] and Bleeker-Rovers and colleagues[13] found that FDG-PET was not helpful if erythrocyte sedimentation rate/CRP was normal.

A few studies have assessed cost.[53,54] Balink and colleagues[53] compared cost in two groups with IUO, one group underwent FDG-PET/CT (n = 46), the other did not (n = 46). A final diagnosis was reached in 70% of patients with FDG-PET/CT compared with only 30% of patients in the other group; costs from diagnostic procedures and hospitalization were lower in the group worked up with FDG-PET/CT because of shorter duration. The authors of both studies concluded that FDG-PET/CT has the potential to become cost-effective in FUO/IUO.

BACTEREMIA

Bacteremia is similar to FUO in that it is systemic in nature with possible infectious sites throughout the body. Nonetheless, several aspects of bacteria in the bloodstream are significantly different; it may lead to metastatic infections through secondary hematogenic spread (eg, prosthetic infections, and spondylodiscitis). Thus, bacteremia can be classified as uncomplicated or metastatic, and morbidity is significantly higher in the latter cases, probably because of insufficient eradication; in uncomplicated bacteremia 2 weeks treatment is usually sufficient, whereas complicated bacteremia with metastatic foci requires several weeks longer. Thus, identification of metastatic infection may have significant clinical impact, but identifying such metastatic infections remains difficult because 50% may be present without signs or symptoms pointing to the areas of interest.[55]

In their landmark study, Vos and colleagues[56,57] prospectively included 115 patients with gram-positive bacteremia to undergo FDG-PET/CT as part of work-up and compared them with a matched historical control group of 230 patients with bacteremia where FDG-PET/CT was not performed. Abnormal findings were verified using a composite reference standard including other imaging, microbiology, or pathology. Results were favorable in several respects, that is, metastatic foci were diagnosed in significantly more cases than control subjects (67.8% vs 35.7%), FDG-PET/CT was the first modality to locate infectious foci in 30% of patients, relapse rate declined from 7.4% in control subjects to 2.6% in cases, and mortality decreased from 32.2% to 19.1%. Based on the same dataset, the same group also assessed cost-effectiveness, and concluded that the impact on morbidity and mortality by introduction of FDG-PET/CT to the routine diagnostic work-up was indeed cost-effective in high-risk patients with gram-positive bacteremia.[58]

Subsequent studies (**Table 3**) have all included some of these aspects while also adding further knowledge, albeit sometimes with different wording. For instance, some studies describe the number of metastatic foci, whereas others present a detection rate for infectious foci, which is in essence just semantics; thus, despite different designation studies find comparable rates for the detection of infectious/metastatic foci, that is, 45.8% to 73.7%.[56,57,59–63] It is noteworthy that Berrevoets and colleagues[59] found 71.2% of the patients with metastatic foci (73.7% of all patients) to be without any signs or symptoms to suggest localization of such foci, and Brøndserud and colleagues[61] corroborated the finding that FDG-PET/

CT is the incremental modality in a significant proportion, that is, 41% (as compared with 30% in the study by Vos and colleagues[56]).

As a supplement to crude diagnostic rate, some studies also assessed the clinical impact on patient management, either changes in treatment or a combination of diagnostic- and treatment-related impact. Thus, Brøndserud and colleagues[61] found "high clinical impact" in 47%, that is, diagnostic findings only present or unequivocal on FDG-PET/CT, establishment of alternative diagnoses, or changes in treatment. Berrevoets and colleagues[59] and Tsai and colleagues[60] only assessed treatment and found FDG-PET/CT to facilitate changes in 74% and 54.1%, respectively, whereas the fraction of treatment changes only constituted 14.7% of the high impact cases in the previously mentioned study by Brøndserud and colleagues.[61] Another approach to personalized treatment based on FDG-PET/CT was presented in another study by the group of Berrevoets and colleagues,[64] that is, 36 cases (bacteremia with high risk of metastatic spread, but negative echocardiography and FDG-PET/CT) treated with antibiotics for the same duration (approximately 15 days) as a control group of patients with uncomplicated bacteremia. Relapse rate and mortality was similar in the two groups suggesting that a shorter course of antibiotics than recommended in complicated bacteremia is safe in cases without signs of metastatic infections.

Several studies have assessed if any parameters impact or predict the diagnostic yield. Tsai and colleagues[60] found that CRP values higher than a cutoff of 54 mg/L resulted in positive findings in 86%, whereas this was the case in only 46% of patients with lower values. The proportion of patients with management changes based on FDG-PET/CT remained comparable (54%). Brøndserud and colleagues[61] found no negative impact on diagnostic yield associated with duration of work-up period or antibiotics before FDG-PET/CT (which could have induced false-negative findings), or underlying malignancies (which could have introduced either false-negative or false-positive findings). However, Pijls and colleagues[62] established a significant negative association between duration of antibiotics before scan and diagnostic yield in univariate and multivariate regression analysis; that is, the overall detection rate was 64.5%, which increased to 71% in patients with less than 7 days antibiotics, whereas it decreased to 52%, 61%, and 38% after 7 to 14 days, 15 to 21 days, and greater than 22 days, respectively.

Table 3
Selected papers on bacteremia

Author (Year)	N	Design	Diagnostic Yield[a]	High Clinical Impact	Change of Treatment	Relapse Rates	Mortality
Vos et al,[56,57] 2010/2012	115 (cases) 230 (control subjects)	Prospective	68% (cases) 36% (control subjects)	N.R.	N.R.	2.6% (cases) 7.4% (control subjects)	19% (cases) 32% (control subjects)
Berrevoets et al,[59] 2017	184	Retrospective	73.7% (DR)	N.R.	74%	N.R.	12.4% (cases) 32.7% (control subjects)
Tsai et al,[60] 2018	102	Retrospective	72.5% (DR)	N.R.	54.1%	N.R.	N.R.
Brøndserud et al,[61] 2019	157	Retrospective	56% (DR)	47%	14.7%	N.R.	N.R.
Pijl et al,[62] 2019	185	Retrospective	64.8% (DR)	N.R.	N.R.	N.R.	N.R.
Yildiz et al,[63] 2019	102	Retrospective	45.8%	N.R.	N.R.	N.R.	16.6% (cases) 44.4% (control subjects)

Abbreviations: DR, detection rate; N.R., not reported.
[a] Either proportion of patients with metastatic infections or overall DR.

Another important parameter is mortality, which Vos and colleagues found positively impacted by FDG-PET/CT, presumably because of higher diagnostic rate of metastatic infections leading to more specific treatment for prolonged periods. Similar results were encountered by Berrevoets and colleagues[59] and Yildiz and colleagues,[63] that is, mortality was reduced from 32.7% (control subjects) to 12.4% (cases), and from 44.4% (control subjects) to 16.6% (cases), respectively.

Limited data are available in pediatrics, but at least one retrospective study found FDG-PET/CT to have potential also in this clinical setting; 13 children with bacteremia and suspected metastatic infection underwent FDG-PET/CT resulting in five true-positives, six true-negatives, two false-positives, and no false-negatives to yield PPV of 71% and NPV of 100%. Thus, the authors concluded that 38% (5/13) was clinically helpful, but again this may be considered conservative because only true-positive findings were considered helpful. If true-negatives are also considered clinically important, FDG-PET/CT could actually be considered helpful in 85% (11/13).[65] Nonetheless, further studies are needed in this particular setting.

FEBRILE NEUTROPENIA

Fever is a frequent finding during the cause of neutropenia in patients with cancer, and because this is a potentially lethal condition, broad-spectrum antibiotics are commonly administered to better patient outcome. However, febrile neutropenia is only caused by infections in 30% to 50% of cases and to avoid significant overtreatment with risk of side effects and resistance induction, it is important to accurately recognize infectious and noninfectious causes of febrile neutropenia.[66] FDG-PET was early suggested as an adjunct to conventional diagnostic work-up,[67] and basic diagnostic yield and clinical impact was the main focus of several studies from the same period (**Table 4**).

Koh and colleagues[68] set up a retrospective case-control cohort based on comparable patients with hematologic malignancies, who developed fever during neutropenic periods and underwent either conventional investigations at the discretion of the managing physician, which included cultures, serology, polymerase chain reaction–based investigations, chest radiograph, and CT in various combinations (control subjects), or conventional investigations and FDG-PET/CT (cases). Final diagnosis was considered infection

Table 4
Selected papers on febrile neutropenia

Author (Year)	N	Design	Underlying Malignancy	Patient Inclusion Criteria	Diagnostic Yield
Vos et al,[66] 2012	28	Prospective	Hematologic malignancies[a]	NC <0.1 × 10/L CRP >50 mg/L	N.R.
Koh et al,[68] 2012	37 (76 control subjects)	Retrospective	Hematologic malignancies	>38.3°C NC <0.5 × 10⁹/L	94.6% (cases)[b] 69.7% (control subjects)[b]
Guy et al,[69] 2012	20	Prospective	Hematologic malignancies (n = 19) Solid tumor (n = 1)	>38°C NC <500 cells/μL	N.R.
Gafter-Gvili et al,[70] 2013	79	Prospective	Hematologic malignancies	Fever NC <500 cells/mm³	80%/32% (FDG-PET/CT)[c] 73%/42% (whole-body CT)[c]
Camus et al,[72] 2015	48	Prospective	Hematologic malignancies	>38°C NC <500 cells/μL	61%/90%[c] PPV 96%
Wang et al,[71] 2018	14	Retrospective	Immunosuppressed children	>38°C NC <0.47 cells/μL	N.R.

Abbreviations: NC, neutrophil count; N.R., not reported.
[a] Either intensive treatment chemotherapy or myeloablative therapy before hematopoietic stem cell transplantation.
[b] Detection rate.
[c] Sensitivity/specificity.

in two-thirds of patients in both groups, but only 5% of cases remained unclarified, whereas this was true for 30% of control subjects; thus, detection rate for underlying disease was 94.6% of cases and 69.7% of control subjects. FDG-PET/CT had significant impact on treatment strategy in one-third of cases compared with an impact of conventional imaging in 1 of 10 control subjects, and duration of systemic antifungal therapy was significantly shorter in cases than control subjects. Comparable results were encountered by Guy and colleagues[69] and Gafter-Gvili and colleagues.[70] In the former, 20 patients underwent conventional imaging and FDG-PET/CT; FDG-PET/CT found infectious foci in seven patients with negative conventional imaging, located eight additional infectious foci in other patients, and FDG-PET/CT were overall considered to have high clinical impact in 75% (ie, location of additional foci or direct impact on therapy).[69] In the latter, FDG-PET/CT generally performed comparably with whole-body CT, but still lead to changed diagnosis or treatment in 69% and 55%, respectively.[70] Similar results were found in a recent study in a pediatric setting, that is, high clinical impact in 79%, and a positive contribution to final diagnosis in 60% of patients.[71] However, the most recent study from 2015 by Camus and colleagues[72] found more equivocal results, that is, a sensitivity of only 61%, albeit with high specificity and PPV, and with no discernible clinical impact on diagnosis or treatment, and the authors conclude that although FDG-PET/CT has potential, they found no advantage over CT. Thus, despite the initial success and potential for lesion detection of FDG-PET/CT in the setting of febrile neutropenia, results remain equivocal and based on small studies with methodologic issues (eg, ill-defined reference standards primarily based on post hoc clinical adjudication often also based on results of FDG-PET/CT). Also, most studies included only hematologic malignancies, whereas the potential value in patients with solid tumors is virtually nonexplored.

Several additional features are worth considering. First, mucosal inflammation in the digestive tract also presents with fever and is an important differential diagnosis, but is also associated with certain pathogens (eg, *Streptococcus mitis*). Second, bacteremia with coagulase-negative staphylococci is commonly associated with central venous catheters but may also be secondary to mucosal inflammation. Third, invasive pulmonary fungal infestation is an important differential cause of bacteremia in febrile neutropenia with high mortality. Thus, Vos and colleagues[66] undertook a prospective observational/descriptive study to establish if FDG-PET/CT provided additional value when it was added to standard work-up in patients with neutropenia with hematologic malignancies and a rise in CRP greater than 50 mg/L (thus, strictly not febrile neutropenia). They found several results with relevance to the previously mentioned special features; that is, FDG uptake in central venous catheters was associated with coagulase-negative staphylococci and deep venous thrombosis, high esophageal FDG-uptake was associated with *S mitis*, and pulmonary FDG uptake was associated with invasive fungal disease. The study was limited by few patients, and a reference standard was not applied routinely.

Some limitations to the use of FDG-PET/CT have been brought forth in febrile neutropenia. Sensitivity could be hampered because FDG uptake in activated neutrophils is considered an essential pathophysiologic basis for positive FDG PET/CT findings in infectious settings, and specificity may be hampered because of the nonspecific uptake in underlying malignancies and metastases. Nonetheless, in reality sensitivity is hardly a challenge; several of the previously mentioned studies report high detection rates even in nonsymptomatic patients.[66,67,69] Older studies have also shown autoradiographically that FDG uptake is present not only in neutrophils but also macrophages and constituents of granulation tissue, which may explain the uptake despite severe neutropenia.[73,74] Regarding specificity, with the increasing use of FDG-PET/CT in the diagnostic work-up or staging of malignancies, the possibility of comparison in suspected infection may help interpretation, and data from several of the previously mentioned studies did not point to specificity issues because they reported only few or no equivocal or false-positive findings.[68,69]

DISCLOSURE

Nothing to disclose.

REFERENCES

1. Mulders-Manders C, Simon A, Bleeker-Rovers C. Fever of unknown origin. Clin Med (Lond) 2015; 15(3):280–4.
2. Petersdorf RG, Beeson PB. Fever of unexplained origin: report on 100 cases. Medicine 1961;40:1–30.
3. Blockmans D, Knockaert D, Maes A, et al. Clinical value of [(18)F]fluoro-deoxyglucose positron emission tomography for patients with fever of unknown origin. Clin Infect Dis 2001;32(2):191–6.

4. Hung BT, Wang PW, Su YJ, et al. The efficacy of (18) F-FDG PET/CT and (67)Ga SPECT/CT in diagnosing fever of unknown origin. Int J Infect Dis 2017;62: 10–7.

5. Kjaer A, Lebech AM, Eigtved A, et al. Fever of unknown origin: prospective comparison of diagnostic value of 18F-FDG PET and 111In-granulocyte scintigraphy. Eur J Nucl Med Mol Imaging 2004;31(5):622–6.

6. Bleeker-Rovers CP, Corstens FH, Van Der Meer JW, et al. Fever of unknown origin: prospective comparison of diagnostic value of (18)F-FDG PET and (111) In-granulocyte scintigraphy. Eur J Nucl Med Mol Imaging 2004;31(9):1342–3 [author reply: 4].

7. Seshadri N, Sonoda LI, Lever AM, et al. Superiority of 18F-FDG PET compared to 111In-labelled leucocyte scintigraphy in the evaluation of fever of unknown origin. J Infect 2012;65(1):71–9.

8. Takeuchi M, Dahabreh IJ, Nihashi T, et al. Nuclear imaging for classic fever of unknown origin: meta-analysis. J Nucl Med 2016;57(12):1913–9.

9. Lorenzen J, Buchert R, Bohuslavizki KH. Value of FDG PET in patients with fever of unknown origin. Nucl Med Commun 2001;22(7):779–83.

10. Bleeker-Rovers CP, de Kleijn EM, Corstens FH, et al. Clinical value of FDG PET in patients with fever of unknown origin and patients suspected of focal infection or inflammation. Eur J Nucl Med Mol Imaging 2004;31(1):29–37.

11. Buysschaert I, Vanderschueren S, Blockmans D, et al. Contribution of (18)fluoro-deoxyglucose positron emission tomography to the work-up of patients with fever of unknown origin. Eur J Intern Med 2004; 15(3):151–6.

12. Jaruskova M, Belohlavek O. Role of FDG-PET and PET/CT in the diagnosis of prolonged febrile states. Eur J Nucl Med Mol Imaging 2006;33(8):913–8.

13. Bleeker-Rovers CP, Vos FJ, Mudde AH, et al. A prospective multi-centre study of the value of FDG-PET as part of a structured diagnostic protocol in patients with fever of unknown origin. Eur J Nucl Med Mol Imaging 2007;34(5):694–703.

14. Vanderschueren S, Del Biondo E, Ruttens D, et al. Inflammation of unknown origin versus fever of unknown origin: two of a kind. Eur J Intern Med 2009; 20(4):415–8.

15. Kubota K, Nakamoto Y, Tamaki N, et al. FDG-PET for the diagnosis of fever of unknown origin: a Japanese multi-center study. Ann Nucl Med 2011;25(5): 355–64.

16. Keidar Z, Gurman-Balbir A, Gaitini D, et al. Fever of unknown origin: the role of 18F-FDG PET/CT. J Nucl Med 2008;49(12):1980–5.

17. Balink H, Collins J, Bruyn GA, et al. F-18 FDG PET/ CT in the diagnosis of fever of unknown origin. Clin Nucl Med 2009;34(12):862–8.

18. Federici L, Blondet C, Imperiale A, et al. Value of (18)F-FDG-PET/CT in patients with fever of unknown origin and unexplained prolonged inflammatory syndrome: a single centre analysis experience. Int J Clin Pract 2010;64(1):55–60.

19. Ferda J, Ferdova E, Zahlava J, et al. Fever of unknown origin: a value of (18)F-FDG-PET/CT with integrated full diagnostic isotropic CT imaging. Eur J Radiol 2010;73(3):518–25.

20. Kei PL, Kok TY, Padhy AK, et al. [18F] FDG PET/ CT in patients with fever of unknown origin: a local experience. Nucl Med Commun 2010;31(9): 788–92.

21. Rosenbaum J, Basu S, Beckerman S, et al. Evaluation of diagnostic performance of 18F-FDG-PET compared to CT in detecting potential causes of fever of unknown origin in an academic centre. Hell J Nucl Med 2011;14(3):255–9.

22. Sheng JF, Sheng ZK, Shen XM, et al. Diagnostic value of fluorine-18 fluorodeoxyglucose positron emission tomography/computed tomography in patients with fever of unknown origin. Eur J Intern Med 2011;22(1):112–6.

23. Pelosi E, Skanjeti A, Penna D, et al. Role of integrated PET/CT with [(1)(8)F]-FDG in the management of patients with fever of unknown origin: a single-centre experience. La Radiologia Med 2011; 116(5):809–20.

24. Ergul N, Halac M, Cermik TF, et al. The diagnostic role of FDG PET/CT in patients with fever of unknown origin. Mol Imaging Radionucl Ther 2011;20(1): 19–25.

25. Crouzet J, Boudousq V, Lechiche C, et al. Place of (18)F-FDG-PET with computed tomography in the diagnostic algorithm of patients with fever of unknown origin. Eur J Clin Microbiol Infect Dis 2012; 31(8):1727–33.

26. Kim YJ, Kim SI, Hong KW, et al. Diagnostic value of 18F-FDG PET/CT in patients with fever of unknown origin. Intern Med J 2012;42(7):834–7.

27. Pedersen TI, Roed C, Knudsen LS, et al. Fever of unknown origin: a retrospective study of 52 cases with evaluation of the diagnostic utility of FDG-PET/CT. Scand J Infect Dis 2012;44(1):18–23.

28. Manohar K, Mittal BR, Jain S, et al. F-18 FDG-PET/ CT in evaluation of patients with fever of unknown origin. Jpn J Radiol 2013;31(5):320–7.

29. Tokmak H, Ergonul O, Demirkol O, et al. Diagnostic contribution of (18)F-FDG-PET/CT in fever of unknown origin. Int J Infect Dis 2014;19:53–8.

30. Buch-Olsen KM, Andersen RV, Hess S, et al. 18F-FDG-PET/CT in fever of unknown origin: clinical value. Nucl Med Commun 2014;35(9): 955–60.

31. Gafter-Gvili A, Raibman S, Grossman A, et al. [18F] FDG-PET/CT for the diagnosis of patients with fever of unknown origin. QJM 2015;108(4):289–98.

32. Bouter C, Braune I, Meller B, et al. (18)F-FDG-PET/CT in unexplained elevated inflammatory

markers. Joining entities. Nuklearmedizin 2016; 55(6):242–9.

33. Schonau V, Vogel K, Englbrecht M, et al. The value of (18)F-FDG-PET/CT in identifying the cause of fever of unknown origin (FUO) and inflammation of unknown origin (IUO): data from a prospective study. Ann Rheum Dis 2018;77(1):70–7.

34. Abdelrahman SF, Elsayed ND, El-nasr SIS, et al. Value of 18-F-FDG PET/CT in assessment of patients with fever of unknown origin. Egypt J Radiol Nucl Med 2018;49(2):461–6.

35. Singh N, Kumar R, Malhotra A, et al. Diagnostic utility of fluorodeoxyglucose positron emission tomography/computed tomography in pyrexia of unknown origin. Indian J Nucl Med 2015;30(3): 204–12.

36. Wang Q, Li YM, Li Y, et al. (18)F-FDGPET/CT in fever of unknown origin and inflammation of unknown origin: a Chinese multi-center study. Eur J Nucl Med Mol Imaging 2019;46(1):159–65.

37. Bleeker-Rovers CP, Vos FJ, de Kleijn EM, et al. A prospective multicenter study on fever of unknown origin: the yield of a structured diagnostic protocol. Medicine 2007;86(1):26–38.

38. Dong MJ, Zhao K, Liu ZF, et al. A meta-analysis of the value of fluorodeoxyglucose-PET/PET-CT in the evaluation of fever of unknown origin. Eur J Radiol 2011;80(3):834–44.

39. Hao R, Yuan L, Kan Y, et al. Diagnostic performance of 18F-FDG PET/CT in patients with fever of unknown origin: a meta-analysis. Nucl Med Commun 2013;34(7):682–8.

40. Kan Y, Wang W, Liu J, et al. Contribution of 18F-FDG PET/CT in a case-mix of fever of unknown origin and inflammation of unknown origin: a meta-analysis. Acta Radiol 2019;60(6):716–25.

41. Besson FL, Chaumet-Riffaud P, Playe M, et al. Contribution of (18)F-FDG PET in the diagnostic assessment of fever of unknown origin (FUO): a stratification-based meta-analysis. Eur J Nucl Med Mol Imaging 2016;43(10):1887–95.

42. Bharucha T, Rutherford A, Skeoch S, et al. Diagnostic yield of FDG-PET/CT in fever of unknown origin: a systematic review, meta-analysis, and Delphi exercise. Clin Radiol 2017;72(9):764–71.

43. Takeuchi M, Nihashi T, Gafter-Gvili A, et al. Association of 18F-FDG PET or PET/CT results with spontaneous remission in classic fever of unknown origin: a systematic review and meta-analysis. Medicine 2018;97(43):e12909.

44. Castaigne C, Tondeur M, de Wit S, et al. Clinical value of FDG-PET/CT for the diagnosis of human immunodeficiency virus-associated fever of unknown origin: a retrospective study. Nucl Med Commun 2009;30(1):41–7.

45. Martin C, Castaigne C, Tondeur M, et al. Role and interpretation of fluorodeoxyglucose-positron emission tomography/computed tomography in HIV-infected patients with fever of unknown origin: a prospective study. HIV Med 2013;14(8):455–62.

46. Simons KS, Pickkers P, Bleeker-Rovers CP, et al. F-18-fluorodeoxyglucose positron emission tomography combined with CT in critically ill patients with suspected infection. Intensive Care Med 2010; 36(3):504–11.

47. Jasper N, Dabritz J, Frosch M, et al. Diagnostic value of [(18)F]-FDG PET/CT in children with fever of unknown origin or unexplained signs of inflammation. Eur J Nucl Med Mol Imaging 2010;37(1): 136–45.

48. Blokhuis GJ, Bleeker-Rovers CP, Diender MG, et al. Diagnostic value of FDG-PET/(CT) in children with fever of unknown origin and unexplained fever during immune suppression. Eur J Nucl Med Mol Imaging 2014;41(10):1916–23.

49. Sturm E, Rings EH, Scholvinck EH, et al. Fluorodeoxyglucose positron emission tomography contributes to management of pediatric liver transplantation candidates with fever of unknown origin. Liver Transpl 2006;12(11):1698–704.

50. Balink H, Veeger NJ, Bennink RJ, et al. The predictive value of C-reactive protein and erythrocyte sedimentation rate for 18F-FDG PET/CT outcome in patients with fever and inflammation of unknown origin. Nucl Med Commun 2015;36(6):604–9.

51. Pereira AM, Husmann L, Sah BR, et al. Determinants of diagnostic performance of 18F-FDG PET/CT in patients with fever of unknown origin. Nucl Med Commun 2016;37(1):57–65.

52. Garcia-Vicente AM, Tello-Galan MJ, Amo-Salas M, et al. Do clinical and laboratory variables have any impact on the diagnostic performance of 18F-FDG PET/CT in patients with fever of unknown origin? Ann Nucl Med 2018;32(2):123–31.

53. Balink H, Tan SS, Veeger NJ, et al. (1)(8)F-FDG PET/CT in inflammation of unknown origin: a cost-effectiveness pilot-study. Eur J Nucl Med Mol Imaging 2015;42(9):1408–13.

54. Becerra Nakayo EM, Garcia Vicente AM, Soriano Castrejon AM, et al. Analysis of cost-effectiveness in the diagnosis of fever of unknown origin and the role of (18)F-FDG PET-CT: a proposal of diagnostic algorithm. Rev Esp Med Nucl Imagen Mol 2012; 31(4):178–86 [in Spanish].

55. Kouijzer IJ, Vos FJ, Bleeker-Rovers CP, et al. Clinical application of FDG-PET/CT in metastatic infections. Q J Nucl Med Mol Imaging 2017;61(2): 232–46.

56. Vos FJ, Bleeker-Rovers CP, Sturm PD, et al. 18F-FDG PET/CT for detection of metastatic infection in gram-positive bacteremia. J Nucl Med 2010; 51(8):1234–40.

57. Vos FJ, Kullberg BJ, Sturm PD, et al. Metastatic infectious disease and clinical outcome in

Staphylococcus aureus and *Streptococcus* species bacteremia. Medicine 2012;91(2):86–94.

58. Vos FJ, Bleeker-Rovers CP, Kullberg BJ, et al. Cost-effectiveness of routine (18)F-FDG PET/CT in high-risk patients with gram-positive bacteremia. J Nucl Med 2011;52(11):1673–8.

59. Berrevoets MAH, Kouijzer IJE, Aarntzen E, et al. (18)F-FDG PET/CT optimizes treatment in staphylococcus aureus bacteremia and is associated with reduced mortality. J Nucl Med 2017;58(9):1504–10.

60. Tsai HY, Lee MH, Wan CH, et al. C-reactive protein levels can predict positive (18)F-FDG PET/CT findings that lead to management changes in patients with bacteremia. J Microbiol Immunol Infect 2018; 51(6):839–46.

61. Brondserud MB, Pedersen C, Rosenvinge FS, et al. Clinical value of FDG-PET/CT in bacteremia of unknown origin with catalase-negative gram-positive cocci or *Staphylococcus aureus*. Eur J Nucl Med Mol Imaging 2019;46(6):1351–8.

62. Pijl JP, Glaudemans A, Slart R, et al. FDG-PET/CT for detecting an infection focus in patients with bloodstream infection: factors affecting diagnostic yield. Clin Nucl Med 2019;44(2):99–106.

63. Yildiz H, Reychler G, Rodriguez-Villalobos H, et al. Mortality in patients with high risk *Staphylococcus aureus* bacteremia undergoing or not PET-CT: a single center experience. J Infect Chemother 2019. https://doi.org/10.1016/j.jiac.2019.04.016.

64. Berrevoets MAH, Kouijzer IJE, Slieker K, et al. (18)F-FDG-PET/CT-guided treatment duration in patients with high-risk *Staphylococcus aureus* bacteremia: a proof of principle. J Nucl Med 2018. https://doi.org/10.2967/jnumed.118.221929.

65. Kouijzer IJ, Blokhuis GJ, Draaisma JM, et al. 18F-FDG PET/CT in detecting metastatic infection in children. Clin Nucl Med 2016;41(4):278–81.

66. Vos FJ, Donnelly JP, Oyen WJG, et al. 18F-FDG PET/CT for diagnosing infectious complications in patients with severe neutropenia after intensive chemotherapy for haematological malignancy or stem cell transplantation. Eur J Nucl Med Mol Imaging 2012;39(1):120–8.

67. Mahfouz T, Miceli MH, Saghafifar F, et al. 18F-fluorodeoxyglucose positron emission tomography contributes to the diagnosis and management of infections in patients with multiple myeloma: a study of 165 infectious episodes. J Clin Oncol 2005;23(31): 7857–63.

68. Koh KC, Slavin MA, Thursky KA, et al. Impact of fluorine-18 fluorodeoxyglucose positron emission tomography on diagnosis and antimicrobial utilization in patients with high-risk febrile neutropenia. Leuk Lymphoma 2012;53(10):1889–95.

69. Guy SD, Tramontana AR, Worth LJ, et al. Use of FDG PET/CT for investigation of febrile neutropenia: evaluation in high-risk cancer patients. Eur J Nucl Med Mol Imaging 2012;39(8):1348–55.

70. Gafter-Gvili A, Paul M, Bernstine H, et al. The role of (1)(8)F-FDG PET/CT for the diagnosis of infections in patients with hematological malignancies and persistent febrile neutropenia. Leuk Res 2013; 37(9):1057–62.

71. Wang SS, Mechinaud F, Thursky K, et al. The clinical utility of fluorodeoxyglucose-positron emission tomography for investigation of fever in immunocompromised children. J Paediatr Child Health 2018; 54(5):487–92.

72. Camus V, Edet-Sanson A, Bubenheim M, et al. (1)(8)F-FDG-PET/CT imaging in patients with febrile neutropenia and haematological malignancies. Anticancer Res 2015;35(5):2999–3005.

73. Kubota R, Yamada S, Kubota K, et al. Intratumoral distribution of fluorine-18-fluorodeoxyglucose in vivo: high accumulation in macrophages and granulation tissues studied by microautoradiography. J Nucl Med 1992;33(11):1972–80.

74. Yamada S, Kubota K, Kubota R, et al. High accumulation of fluorine-18-fluorodeoxyglucose in turpentine-induced inflammatory tissue. J Nucl Med 1995;36(7):1301–6.

75. Schönau V, Vogel K, Englbrecht M, et al. The value of 18F-FDG-PET/CT in identifying the cause of fever of unknown origin (FUO) and inflammation of unknown origin (IUO): data from a prospective study. Ann Rheum Dis 2018;77(1):70–7. https://doi.org/10.1136/annrheumdis-2017-211687. Epub 2017 Sep 19.

18F-Fluorodeoxyglucose PET/Computed Tomography in Endocarditis

Asbjørn Mathias Scholtens, MD

KEYWORDS

- Endocarditis • Infection • Prosthetic heart valves • Cardiac implantable electronic devices • Grafts
- Left ventricular assist devices • FDG-PET/CT

KEY POINTS

- The role of 18F-fluorodeoxyglucose (FDG) PET/computed tomography (CT) in the diagnosis of endocarditis and implant infection.
- Current evidence for FDG-PET/CT in the diagnosis of endocarditis and implant infection.
- Recommendations for acquisition, (semi)quantification, and interpretation of FDG-PET/CT studies performed in the context of possible cardiac infections.

INTRODUCTION

Infection of the heart predominantly takes the form of endocarditis, infection of the inner lining of the heart, most notably the valves. Prosthetic materials such as valve replacements, grafts, implantable devices, and their associated materials such as leads are predisposing factors for developing endocarditis. The initial presentation of endocarditis is diverse, with few symptoms specific for the disease, making the initial diagnosis challenging. Echocardiography is the first line of imaging, with excellent accuracy in native valve imaging, but it may be hampered by acoustic shadowing and reverberation when imaging implanted material. The potential for additional value of other imaging techniques is high, and in recent years both the interest in and the evidence for 18F-fluorodeoxyglucose (FDG) PET/computed tomography (CT) in this complex diagnosis has expanded significantly.

The role of FDG-PET/CT in infections of the heart has been reviewed in detail by Millar and colleagues[1] in a recent edition of *PET Clinics*; in the current article, the general concepts and available evidence are reviewed with a focus on recent publications, and recommendations for image acquisition and interpretation are given.

PATIENT PREPARATION

As described in more detail in the article by Søren Hess and colleagues, "Patient Preparation and Patient Related Challenges in Infectious and Inflammatory Disease," in this issue, patient preparation for FDG-PET/CT is especially important when evaluating the heart and its surrounding tissues. Unlike most other surrounding tissues, myocardial glucose consumption is highly variable and depends on the overall metabolic state of the patient, mediated by glucose transporter (GLUT) type 4. Myocardial glucose uptake increases when glucose serum availability and/or insulin levels are high, and decreases when insulin levels are low and free fatty acid (FFA) levels are high in concordance with the Randle cycle. Inflammatory cell glucose consumption is regulated by GLUT1 and GLUT3 and is essentially independent from the overall metabolic state.

Although many protocols for patient preparation have been described in the literature,[2] there is no definite consensus on the most appropriate protocol as of this writing. Recent publications,[3,4] including the most recent Japanese Society of Nuclear Cardiology recommendations,[5] agree that low-carbohydrate fat-allowed diets and prolonged

Meander Medical Center, Nuclear Medicine, Afd.Nucleaire Geneeskunde, Maatweg 3, Amersfoort 3813TZ, the Netherlands
E-mail address: a.scholtens@meandermc.nl

PET Clin 15 (2020) 187–195
https://doi.org/10.1016/j.cpet.2019.11.003
1556-8598/20/© 2019 Elsevier Inc. All rights reserved.

fasting are cornerstones of current preparatory protocols, but there is still debate regarding the added value of unfractionated heparin bolus infusion to increase FFA serum levels. In our experience, heparin functions as an adjunct to diet and fasting, increasing the suppression of myocardial glucose metabolism.[6]

PROSTHETIC HEART VALVE ENDOCARDITIS

The largest amount of evidence for the use of FDG-PET/CT in cardiac infection is available for prosthetic heart valve endocarditis (PVE). The seminal article by Saby and colleagues[7] showed good sensitivity of 73% and specificity of 80% for FDG-PET/CT in a cohort of 72 patients, and, when added to the Duke criteria, increased sensitivity from 70% to 93%. Since then, numerous publications have addressed the added value of FDG-PET/CT in the setting of PVE, and a meta-analysis by Mahmood and colleagues[8] of single-center data published between 2013 and 2017 calculated a pooled sensitivity of 80.5% and specificity of 73.1%. In 2018, analysis of a large, retrospective, multicenter cohort showed a sensitivity of 74% and specificity of 91% but also identified significant confounders in the form of low inflammatory activity, defined as a C-reactive protein level less than 40 and the use of surgical adhesive during implantation (false-negative and false-positive confounders, respectively), and exclusion of these confounders increased the sensitivity and specificity of FDG-PET/CT in PVE to 91% and 95%.[9] In 2019, a large, single center cohort of 188 patients with suspicion of left-sided PVE reported a sensitivity of 93% and a specificity of 90%.[10]

NATIVE VALVE ENDOCARDITIS

In native valve endocarditis (NVE), FDG-PET/CT has a far lower sensitivity than in PVE, with a recent study with a large cohort of 115 patients with suspected NVE reporting a sensitivity of only 22%.[10] Although specificity is high, the diagnostic accuracy for valve infection is low. A likely explanation is the initial presentation of NVE, which in most cases involves vegetations on valve leaflets. Such vegetations are generally small and, perhaps more importantly, have been shown to elicit very little white blood cell response even when colonized with bacteria. Because FDG-PET/CT depends on white blood cell migration and glucose consumption to elicit a signal, the likelihood of detection decreases. A recent publication showed lower polymorphonuclear cell involvement and higher fibrosis in NVE compared with PVE in

pathology reports.[10] As such, positive FDG-PET/CT findings in NVE may indicate a more complicated infection with involvement of perivalvular structures, although no definite conclusion can be drawn based on the current evidence. Nevertheless, current literature does suggest that FDG-PET/CT findings of probable infectious emboli and other infectious foci have additional value in NVE, with metastatic foci found in up to 55% of patients.[11]

CARDIAC IMPLANTABLE ELECTRONIC DEVICE INFECTION

The role of FDG-PET/CT in cardiac implantable electronic device infection (CIEDI) has seen an increasing amount of interest in recent years, much like in PVE. A meta-analysis from 2019 that included 14 studies reported a sensitivity of 83% and specificity of 89%.[12] FDG-PET/CT was better equipped to diagnose pocket infection (sensitivity 96%, specificity 97%) than to diagnose lead infection (sensitivity 76%, specificity 83%). Of note, FDG-PET/CT was performed after special dietary preparation in only 4 of the included studies, and physiologic myocardial uptake of FDG may therefore have hampered the interpretation of the cardiac portion of the leads in the other studies. Another possible explanation for the lower accuracy in lead infection may be that small lead vegetations, much like valve vegetations, may not elicit much leukocyte response and may thus be underdiagnosed. In addition, many patients had already been treated with antibiotic therapy.

A recent study including 105 patients with the clinical suspicion of CIEDI showed FDG-PET/CT reclassified nearly 1 in 4 patients when added to the modified Duke criteria, and after including the PET findings the criteria showed a significant difference in survival between definite CIEDI-related endocarditis and the possible/rejected subgroups.[13]

LEFT VENTRICULAR ASSIST DEVICE INFECTION

Left ventricular assist devices (LVADs) are essentially implantable pumps that perform the circulatory function for the heart. They typically consist of a percutaneous driveline to the pump that is connected to the circulation via an inflow cannula through the left ventricle apex and an outflow cannula connected to the ascending aorta. Because it is the only part to percutaneously remain in contact with the outside world, the driveline is especially at risk of infection.

A recent case series and meta-analysis of 4 articles on FDG-PET/CT in LVAD infection published in July 2019 showed a pooled sensitivity of 92% and specificity of 83% for the detection of LVAD infection, noting that specificity differed over a large range between the studies (25%–100%).[14] In a comparison between FDG-PET/CT and labeled-leukocyte scintigraphy, the sensitivity of FDG-PET/CT was significantly higher (95% vs 71%) and it should be considered as the first-line nuclear imaging test in LVAD infection.[15]

A potential reason for false-positive findings, much like in PVE, is the use of surgical adhesives to reinforce the inflow and outflow cannulas. As written in an article on techniques for LVAD placement in 2011, surgeons "are not above application of glues to the aortic suture line and the apical connection"[16] but this is not necessarily standard procedure, and availability of the surgical report of the implantation procedure can make a great difference in the interpretation of findings. In addition, the large, dense structures of the pump housing are especially prone to beam hardening and scatter on the low-dose CT images used for attenuation correction (AC), leading to false increased signal on the AC PET/CT images.

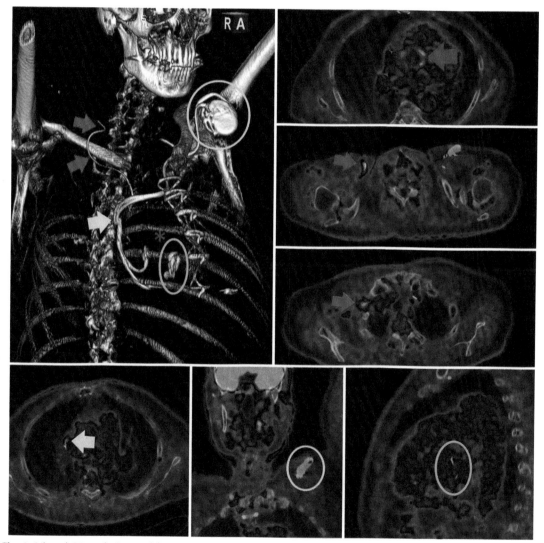

Fig. 1. Virtual CT rendering and fused PET/CT images in this patient with an intracardiac defibrillator, a prosthetic mitral valve replacement, and a homograft replacement of the aortic valve and ascending aorta show increased metabolic activity associated with confirmed infection surrounding the homograft (*red arrow and asterisk*), in 2 foci on the intravenous access cannula in the right jugular vein (*orange arrows*), and in a focus on the implantable cardioverter-defibrillator (ICD) leads in the vena cava (*yellow arrows*). There are no signs of infection near the ICD pocket (*blue circles*) or the prosthetic mitral valve (*green ellipses*).

VALUE OF MULTIMODALITY IMAGING

Although FDG-PET/CT can identify infection before anatomic damage has occurred, it is not the ideal modality to assess whether damage has occurred. In addition, as explained earlier, vegetations cannot be effectively ruled out with FDG-PET/CT alone. Although it is standard practice to perform echocardiography on all patients suspected of endocarditis, which is generally highly effective in diagnosing NVE, both transthoracic echocardiography (TTE) and transesophageal echocardiography (TEE) may have difficulties when devices or prosthetic valves are involved because of acoustic shadowing. Cardiac-triggered CT angiography (CTA) has been shown to be of additional value, increasing sensitivity and specificity from 86.4% and 87.5% for FDG-PET/CT to 91% and 90.6% for FDG-PET/CTA, respectively.[17] In a recent study in which the flowchart included echocardiography, CTA, and FDG-PET/CT in a mixed population including NVE, PVE, CIEDI, and LVAD infection, 73% of cases were identified by echocardiography, 68% by multidetector CTA, 63% by FDG-PET/CT, and 95% by all techniques together.[18]

It is important to realize that all imaging modalities come with their own strengths and weaknesses, and, in the difficult setting of device infection and/or PVE, multimodality imaging is

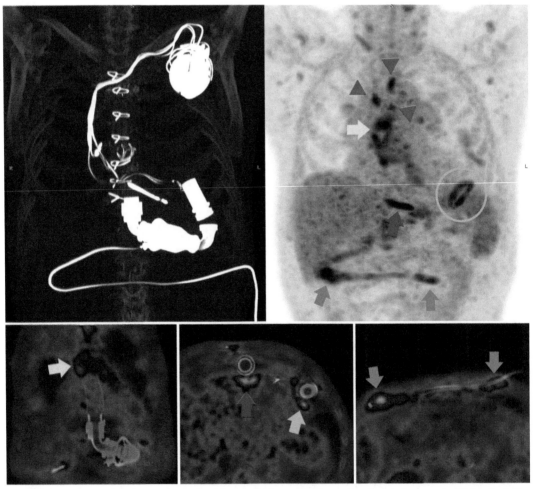

Fig. 2. FDG-PET/CT in a febrile patient with a history of bioprosthetic aortic valve replacement, ICD implantation, and LVAD implantation. There are multiple areas of increased metabolic activity around the LVAD, indicating infection: at the anastomosis of the outflow cannula with the ascending aorta (*yellow arrows*), near the outflow portion of the pump housing (*red arrows*), and heterogeneously along the driveline (*blue arrows*). Multiple active lymph nodes in the mediastinum further support the diagnosis of infection (*orange arrowheads*). The circular uptake near the inflow cannula at the apex of the heart (*green arrow and circle*) may be caused by surgical adhesives applied there according to the surgical report. There is no activity near the ICD or its leads, or near the prosthetic heart valve.

especially valuable and should be evaluated in a multidisciplinary setting (commonly referred to as an endocarditis team) including cardiologists, microbiologists, radiologists, and nuclear medicine physicians.[19]

IMAGE ACQUISITION

Total body imaging is the preferred protocol to rule out infectious foci in the extremities. Although the visualization of intracranial lesions is difficult because of the physiologically high uptake of FDG in the brain, larger lesions may be visible even in this background.

Additional gated images of the cardiac region may be of additional value by visualizing cardiac and valve motion through the cardiac cycle, and may be more easily compared with CTA images. However, this does entail an added scan time burden for the patient, whereas no publications to date have addressed the added value of gated imaging in the diagnostic accuracy of FDG-PET/CT in endocarditis, so no clear recommendation can be given.

Late imaging has been proposed in case studies[20,21] based on the fact that physiologic background activity in the blood pool diminishes over time and lesions will be more readily identified. This property may be of additional value in CIEDI, particularly to address lead infection, for which sensitivity is lower. However, a patient series reporting a comparison between imaging 60 minutes and 150 minutes postinjection found a propensity for false-positive interpretation of the late images in the setting of PVE, and such images must be read with caution.[22]

In the current European Society of Cardiology guidelines, use of FDG-PET/CT in the first 3 months after surgery is discouraged based on the assumption that false-positive findings may occur because of inflammation related to the healing process.[23] Since then it has become apparent that there is no evidence to support this recommendation, and imaging earlier after surgery does not lead to false-positive interpretation as was originally feared.[9,24,25]

INTERPRETATION

In general, the strongest predictor of infection is focal uptake of FDG in areas where it is not physiologically found; namely in or near valve leaflets, valve annuli, or prosthetic material. In contrast, mild diffuse uptake near mechanical prosthetic

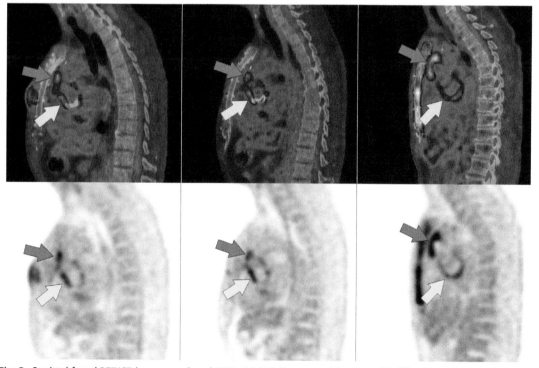

Fig. 3. Sagittal fused PET/CT (*upper row*) and EARL AC PET (*lower row*) images of 3 different patients with Bentall prostheses and documented use of surgical adhesives during implantation. Note the recurring pattern of uptake near the upper anastomosis of the graft (*blue arrows*) and near the lower anastomosis with the aortic valve mechanoprosthesis (*yellow arrows*) corresponding with the administration of adhesive.

Table 1
Potential confounders

Potential Confounder	NVE	PVE	AGI	CIEDI	LVADI
			Effect in:		
Vegetation with low leukocyte infiltration	False-negative. Other imaging modality (TTE/TEE/CTA) needed to rule out vegetation. Important factor for low sensitivity of FDG-PET/CT in this setting	False-negative. Other imaging modality (TTE/TEE/CTA) needed to rule out vegetation	Usually not affected	False-negative, especially with regard to lead infection. Other imaging modality (TTE/TEE/CTA) needed to rule out vegetation	Usually less affected. Vegetation/thrombus inside the LVAD may be visualized by CTA
Surgical adhesives (eg, BioGlue)	Not affected	False-positive. If possible, compare with surgical report	False-positive. If possible, compare with surgical report and/or pattern recognition (see Fig. 3)	Not affected	False-positive. If possible, compare with surgical report
AC artifacts	Not affected	False-positive. Compare with NAC images and consider MAR-algorithm reconstructions	Usually not affected	False-positive. Compare with NAC images and consider MAR-algorithm reconstructions	False-positive. Compare with NAC images and consider MAR-algorithm reconstructions
Noninfectious/physiologic uptake patterns surrounding implanted material	Not affected	Mild diffuse uptake surrounding prosthetic heart valves is a normal variant	Usually not affected. Minor diffuse uptake surrounding the graft may be a normal variant	Not affected	Usually not affected. Mild uptake near pledgeted sutures may be a normal variant
Crista terminalis (muscular ridge in the right atrium, may show uptake of FDG as a physiologic variant)	Not affected	Not affected	Not affected	False-positive if directly adjacent to intra-atrial portions of leads	Not affected
Atrial uptake; eg, in atrial fibrillation	Usually not affected	Usually not affected	Usually not affected	May hamper interpretability of intra-atrial portions of leads	Usually not affected

Potential pitfall				
Lipomatous hypertrophy of the interatrial septum (may show uptake of FDG, likely brown fat). Typical dumbbell-shape on low-dose CT	Possible false-positive caused by proximity to aortic valve	Not affected	Usually not affected	Not affected
Inadequate suppression of physiologic myocardial glucose consumption	Hampers interpretability of infectious activity in intracardiac and paracardiac regions			
Low inflammatory activity (low CRP); eg, caused by prolonged adequate antibiotic therapy	False-negative for the presence of infection			

Abbreviations: AGI, aortic graft infection; CRP, C-reactive protein; LVADI, left ventricular assist device infection; MAR, metal artifact reduction.

valves should be read as a normal variant. In bio-prosthetic valves, some uptake near the valve struts where the leaflets are attached is also a normal variant; although technically multifocal (3 separate foci near the 3 struts), it should be considered a variant of diffuse uptake, especially when mild in intensity.

Intense uptake surrounding prosthetic valves, especially in clinically high suspicion of infection and the absence of other infectious foci, should be interpreted as possible infection even if diffuse.

In patients with aortic grafts, the use of surgical adhesives is more common than in other implants and should be considered if areas of high uptake are confined to the upper and lower edges of the implant and/or near the insertion of the coronaries into the graft, because these are the areas where adhesives are most commonly applied. If possible, the use of adhesives should be confirmed in the surgical report. If the report is unavailable, the possibility of surgical adhesive use should be noted in the differential diagnosis.

No uptake of FDG in the cardiac region should be reported as no evidence of endocarditis, with the caveat that FDG-PET/CT cannot rule out vegetations. However, identification of FDG-avid metastatic infection such as septic lung emboli for right-sided disease and mycotic aneurysms in the extremities or brain abscess for left-sided disease may be considered additional evidence of endocarditis even if there are no cardiac abnormalities. This advice holds especially true in the context of NVE and (to a lesser extent) lead endocarditis, where the sensitivity of FDG-PET/CT is known to be lower for the primary focus, as mentioned earlier. In contrast, if imaging is performed when inflammatory activity is low or has diminished significantly (eg, after adequate antibiotic therapy), readers should be aware of the potential for false-negative results of FDG-PET/CT.

AC artifacts may arise when structures of high density create beam hardening or scatter artifacts on the low-dose CT used for AC. Essentially, non–attenuation-corrected (NAC) images should always be compared with the AC images to exclude such artifacts.

Figs. 1 and **2** show examples in patients with multiple implants. **Fig. 3** shows examples of false-positive FDG uptake related to surgical adhesives. **Table 1** contains an overview of potential confounders in FDG-PET/CT imaging of endocarditis.

FUTURE PERSPECTIVES

The most pressing concern to make FDG-PET/CT more generally applicable in endocarditis is the development of a guideline regarding the standardized reading, interpretation, measurement, and reporting of this modality. In addition, the use of (semi)quantification is hampered by the inability to compare values from different centers unless standardization such as the European Association of Nuclear Medicine Research Ltd (EARL) accreditation has been applied.[26] Because the optimal acquisition and interpretation criteria may differ between native valves and prosthetic materials, and between the different prosthesis types, it is likely that specific guidelines for PVE, CIEDI, and LVAD infection are necessary to ensure enough detail.

SUMMARY

FDG-PET/CT is a valuable tool in the diagnosis of endocarditis, especially in the setting of infection of prosthetic materials. Adequate knowledge of physiologic variants and possible confounders is key in the correct interpretation of FDG-PET/CT findings.

REFERENCES

1. Millar BC, de Camargo RA, Alavi A, et al. PET/Computed tomography evaluation of infection of the heart. PET Clin 2019;14(2):251–69.
2. Osborne MT, Hulten EA, Murthy VL, et al. Patient preparation for cardiac fluorine-18 fluorodeoxyglucose positron emission tomography imaging of inflammation. J Nucl Cardiol 2017;24(1):86–99.
3. Larson SR, Pieper JA, Hulten EA, et al. Characterization of a highly effective preparation for suppression of myocardial glucose utilization. J Nucl Cardiol 2019. [Epub ahead of print].
4. Christopoulos G, Jouni H, Acharya GA, et al. Suppressing physiologic 18-fluorodeoxyglucose uptake in patients undergoing positron emission tomography for cardiac sarcoidosis: the effect of a structured patient preparation protocol. J Nucl Cardiol 2019. [Epub ahead of print].
5. Kumita S, Yoshinaga K, Miyagawa M, et al. Recommendations for (18)F-fluorodeoxyglucose positron emission tomography imaging for diagnosis of cardiac sarcoidosis-2018 update: Japanese Society of Nuclear Cardiology recommendations. J Nucl Cardiol 2019;26(4):1414–33.
6. Scholtens AM, Verberne HJ, Budde RP, et al. Additional heparin preadministration improves cardiac glucose metabolism suppression over low-carbohydrate diet alone in (18)F-FDG PET imaging. J Nucl Med 2016;57(4):568–73.
7. Saby L, Laas O, Habib G, et al. Positron emission tomography/computed tomography for diagnosis of prosthetic valve endocarditis: increased valvular

18F-fluorodeoxyglucose uptake as a novel major criterion. J Am Coll Cardiol 2013;61(23):2374–82.

8. Mahmood M, Kendi AT, Ajmal S, et al. Meta-analysis of 18F-FDG PET/CT in the diagnosis of infective endocarditis. J Nucl Cardiol 2017;26(3):922–35.

9. Swart LE, Gomes A, Scholtens AM, et al. Improving the diagnostic performance of (18)F-fluorodeoxyglucose positron-emission tomography/computed tomography in prosthetic heart valve endocarditis. Circulation 2018;138(14):1412–27.

10. de Camargo RA, Bitencourt MS, Meneghetti JC, et al. The role of 18F-FDG-PET/CT in the Diagnosis of left-sided Endocarditis: native vs. prosthetic valves endocarditis. Clin Infect Dis 2019 [pii: ciz267] [Epub ahead of print].

11. Kouijzer IJE, Berrevoets MAH, Aarntzen EHJG, et al. 18F-fluorodeoxyglucose positron-emission tomography combined with computed tomography as a diagnostic tool in native valve endocarditis. Nucl Med Commun 2018;39(8):747–52.

12. Mahmood M, Kendi AT, Farid S, et al. Role of (18)F-FDG PET/CT in the diagnosis of cardiovascular implantable electronic device infections: a meta-analysis. J Nucl Cardiol 2019;26(3):958–70.

13. Diemberger I, Bonfiglioli R, Martignani C, et al. Contribution of PET imaging to mortality risk stratification in candidates to lead extraction for pacemaker or defibrillator infection: a prospective single center study. Eur J Nucl Med Mol Imaging 2019; 46(1):194–205.

14. Tam MC, Patel VN, Weinberg RL, et al. Diagnostic accuracy of FDG PET/CT in suspected LVAD infections: a case series, systematic review, and meta-analysis. JACC Cardiovasc Imaging 2019 [pii: S1936-878X(19)30568-6]. [Epub ahead of print].

15. de Vaugelade C, Mesguich C, Nubret K, et al. Infections in patients using ventricular-assist devices: comparison of the diagnostic performance of (18) F-FDG PET/CT scan and leucocyte-labeled scintigraphy. J Nucl Cardiol 2019;26(1):42–55.

16. Elefteriades JA, Botta DM Jr. Avoiding technical pitfalls in left ventricular assist device placement. Cardiol Clin 2011;29(4):507–14.

17. Pizzi MN, Roque A, Fernandez-Hidalgo N, et al. Improving the diagnosis of infective endocarditis in prosthetic valves and intracardiac devices with 18F-Fluordeoxyglucose positron emission tomography/computed tomography angiography: initial results at an infective endocarditis referral center. Circulation 2015;132(12):1113–26.

18. Gomes A, van Geel PP, Santing M, et al. Imaging infective endocarditis: adherence to a diagnostic flowchart and direct comparison of imaging techniques. J Nucl Cardiol 2018. [Epub ahead of print].

19. Hyafil F, Rouzet F, Le Guludec D. Nuclear imaging for patients with a suspicion of infective endocarditis: Be part of the team! J Nucl Cardiol 2017;24(1): 207–11.

20. Caldarella C, Leccisotti L, Treglia G, et al. Which is the optimal acquisition time for FDG PET/CT imaging in patients with infective endocarditis? J Nucl Cardiol 2013;20(2):307–9.

21. Leccisotti L, Perna F, Lago M, et al. Cardiovascular implantable electronic device infection: delayed vs standard FDG PET-CT imaging. J Nucl Cardiol 2014;21(3):622–32.

22. Scholtens AM, Swart LE, Verberne HJ, et al. Dual-time-point FDG PET/CT imaging in prosthetic heart valve endocarditis. J Nucl Cardiol 2018;25(6): 1960–7.

23. Authors/Task Force Members, Habib G, Lancellotti P, Antunes MJ, et al. 2015 ESC guidelines for the management of infective endocarditis: the task Force for the management of infective endocarditis of the European Society of Cardiology (ESC)endorsed by: European Association for Cardio-Thoracic Surgery (EACTS), the European Association of Nuclear Medicine (EANM). Eur Heart J 2015;36(44):3075–128.

24. Mathieu C, Mikail N, Benali K, et al. Characterization of 18F-fluorodeoxyglucose uptake pattern in noninfected prosthetic heart valves. Circ Cardiovasc Imaging 2017;10(3):e005585.

25. Scholtens AM, Budde RPJ, Lam MGEH, et al. FDG PET/CT in prosthetic heart valve endocarditis: there is no need to wait. J Nucl Cardiol 2017;24(5): 1540–1.

26. Scholtens AM, Swart LE, Kolste HJT, et al. Standardized uptake values in FDG PET/CT for prosthetic heart valve endocarditis: a call for standardization. J Nucl Cardiol 2017;25(6):2084–91.

18F-FDG PET for Diagnosing Infections in Prosthetic Joints

Robert M. Kwee, MD, PhD[a], Thomas C. Kwee, MD, PhD[b],*

KEYWORDS

- 18F-FDG PET • Positron emission tomography • Joint • Prosthesis • Infection

KEY POINTS

- The diagnostic performance of fludeoxyglucose F 18 (18F-FDG) positron emission tomography (PET) in detecting periprosthetic joint infection (PJI) in hip and knee replacements seems sufficiently high for routine clinical application and adds to conventional tests in terms of diagnostic accuracy.
- Iterative metal artifact reduction of computed tomography data improves PET image quality around prostheses.
- Location rather than intensity of 18F-FDG uptake is critical in diagnosing hip and knee PJI.
- 18F-FDG uptake at the middle portion of the femoral shaft at the bone-prosthesis interface is highly suspicious for hip PJI.
- 18F-FDG uptake at the bone-prosthesis interface has been consistently reported as diagnostic criterion for knee PJI.

INTRODUCTION

In 2010, a little more than 2% of the US population were living with a hip or total knee replacement, which corresponds to approximately 7 million people.[1] Given the increasing number of individuals who choose elective joint replacements to maintain active lifestyles[2] and increasing life expectancy of the general population, the prevalence of hip and knee replacements will continue to increase. Hip and knee replacements can improve function and quality of life of individuals with severe arthritis.[1,3] A major disadvantage, however, is that approximately 6% of all hip and knee replacements need to be revised after 5 years, which rises to as many as 12% after 10 years.[4] More than 25% of revisions are attributed to periprosthetic joint infection (PJI), which is a severe complication and associated with substantial morbidity[5] and high costs.[6,7] Other causes for revisions are polyethylene wear and aseptic loosening, fractures, and dislocations. Whereas fractures and dislocations can readily be distinguished by radiography or computed tomography (CT), it may be difficult to differentiate PJI from aseptic loosening. Accurate preoperative diagnosis of PJI is highly desirable, however, because it determines the method of treatment. Aseptic loosening is treated in a 1-stage revision procedure (prosthesis removal and direct implantation of a new prosthesis), whereas a 2-stage revision procedure (prosthesis removal and delayed reimplantation of a new prosthesis)[5] is considered the current gold standard treatment of PJI.[8]

PATHOGENESIS OF PERIPROSTHETIC JOINT INFECTION

A majority of PJIs occurring within 1 year of surgery are caused by introduction of bacteria at the

[a] Department of Radiology, Zuyderland Medical Center, Heerlen/Sittard/Geleen, The Netherlands;
[b] Department of Radiology, Nuclear Medicine and Molecular Imaging, University Medical Center Groningen, University of Groningen, Hanzeplein 1, PO Box 30.001, Groningen 9700 RB, the Netherlands
* Corresponding author.
E-mail address: thomaskwee@gmail.com

PET Clin 15 (2020) 197–205
https://doi.org/10.1016/j.cpet.2019.11.005
1556-8598/20/© 2019 The Author(s). Published by Elsevier Inc.

time of prosthesis placement, which can occur either through direct contact or aerosolized contamination.[9] Once in contact, bacteria colonize the prosthetic surface.[9] Contiguous spread from an adjacent site is the second mechanism by which PJI can be initiated. This can occur either in the early postoperative period (spread of superficial surgical site infection through incompletely healed superficial and deep fascial planes) or also many years postoperatively (if the normal tissue plane is disrupted again by trauma or surgery).[9] The third mechanism, although less frequent, is hematogeneous spread from a remote infection site.[9] Biofilms are complex communities of bacteria embedded in a protective extracellular matrix that forms on prosthetic surfaces.[9,10] Their formation is intrinsic to the pathogenesis of chronic PJI and is beneficial to bacterial survival and antibiotic resistance.[9–11]

DEFINITION OF PERIPROSTHETIC JOINT INFECTION

In 2018, an updated evidence-based and validated definition for PJI was published.[12] This definition is based on major and minor criteria[12] (**Table 1**). Major criteria include 2 positive cultures or the presence of a sinus tract.[12] Minor criteria include results from preoperative serum and synovial fluid analysis.[12] For patients with inconclusive minor criteria, operative criteria can be used to fulfill the definition of PJI.[12]

DIAGNOSIS OF PERIPROSTHETIC JOINT INFECTION

The typical clinical presentation of PJI is a patient with a painful, warm, stiff, and swollen joint. Clinical presentation, however, frequently is atypical, especially in chronic and low-grade infections, and there are no clinical signs that achieve both high sensitivity and high specificity in diagnosing PJI. A painful joint is the most sensitive but least specific clinical finding in PJI.[11] Signs of deep tissue involvement (ie, sinus tract, purulence, abscess, and extensive necrosis) are the most specific signs and, when present, justify the condition of major criteria for the diagnosis of PJI.[11,12] Clinical findings differ based on the type of joint involved (hip or knee) as well as on the timing and presentation of PJI (ie, early postoperative, acute hematogenous, and chronic).[11] Preoperative synovial fluid culture and serum and synovial fluid analysis for infection markers may be helpful to rule in or rule out PJI (see **Table 1**). An important limitation, however, is the considerable percentage of dry taps, that is, cases in which no fluid can be aspirated despite appropriate anatomic location within the prosthetic hip or knee joint capsule. This percentage has been reported to be as high as 23% and it does not imply that PJI is not present.[13] Other limitations of synovial fluid culture are false-negative results when bacteria are embedded in a biofilm[10] and false-positive cultures when synovial fluid samples are contaminated. Even when using the updated

Table 1
Proposed scoring-based definition for periprosthetic joint infection

Major Criteria (at Least One)			Decision
Two positive cultures of the same organism			Infected
Sinus tract with evidence of communication to the joint or visualization of the prosthesis			

Minor Criteria, Preoperative		Score	Decision
Serum	Elevated CRP or D-dimer	2	≥6 infected
	Elevated ESR	1	2–5 possibly infected
Synovial	Elevated white blood cell count or leukocyte esterase	3	0–1 not infected
	Positive α-defensin	3	
	Elevated polymorphonuclear	2	
	Elevated CRP	1	

Operative Criteria[a]	Score		Decision
Preoperative score	—		≥6 infected
Positive histology	3		4–5 inconclusive
Positive purulence	3		≤3 not infected
Single positive culture	2		

[a] For patients with inconclusive minor criteria.

Adapted from Parvizi J, Tan TL, Goswami K, et al. The 2018 Definition of Periprosthetic Hip and Knee Infection: An Evidence-Based and Validated Criteria. J Arthroplasty. 2018 May;33(5):1309-1314.e2. https://doi.org/10.1016/j.arth.2018.02.078. Epub 2018 Feb 26; with permission.

evidence-based and validated major and minor criteria for PJI,[12] there are patients in whom a diagnosis of PJI cannot be established with certainty preoperatively.[12] Moreover, there are conditions (adverse local tissue reaction, crystalline deposition arthropathy, inflammatory arthropathy flare, and infection with slowly growing organisms [such as *Propionibacterium acnes* and coagulase-negative Staphylococci]) in which the criteria may be inaccurate.[12]

ROLE OF IMAGING, INCLUDING FLUDEOXYGLUCOSE F 18 POSITRON EMISSION TOMOGRAPHY

The diagnostic approach in patients with suspected PJI is variable from center to center.[14] It depends on local experience and availability of technological equipment.[14] Also, there currently are no published evidence-based guidelines to guide the diagnostic work-up of PJI.[14] **Table 2** provides a global, descriptive overview of the accuracy of different imaging modalities.

Radiography usually is the initial imaging modality to evaluate possible PJI.[5,15] Its sensitivity and specificity are low: osteolysis and periosteal reaction are late findings and also may occur in aseptic loosening.[5,15] CT[16] and magnetic resonance imaging (MRI) using metal artifact reduction sequences may be more accurate, because they can detect soft tissue abnormalities associated with PJI, included among which are periarticular fluid collections, joint effusion, synovitis, lymphadenopathy, and sinus tracts.[17–19] The accuracy of these cross-sectional imaging modalities, however, has not yet been widely validated. Granulomatous reactions to wear, the concurrence of adverse local tissue reaction and PJI, and

underlying rheumatoid diseases may impede assessment by CT and MRI.[17]

There are several nuclear imaging techniques that can be used to evaluate suspected PJI. Bone scintigraphy with technetium Tc 99m (^{99m}Tc)-labeled diphosphonates or, alternatively, sodium fluoride F 18 PET[20] can be used to assess osteoblastic activity around the prosthesis. Because sensitivity is high,[21,22] normal findings can be considered strong evidence against the presence of PJI.[23] Specificity, however, generally is low[21,22]; positive findings can indicate either PJI or aseptic loosening. Moreover, a bone scan may be positive for at least 2 years after hip replacement and at least 5 years after knee replacement due to physiologic bone remodeling.[23] Because bone scintigraphy with ^{99m}Tc-labeled diphosphonates is relatively cheap, it may be used as an initial screening test for suspected PJI. Labeled leukocyte imaging has shown superior accuracy for diagnosing PJI compared with bone scintigraphy.[21,22] A caveat, however, is the normal physiologic accumulation of white blood cells in the bone marrow, which may be variable from 1 person to another.[23] Furthermore, hematopoietically active marrow usually develops around joint prostheses, producing an alteration of the normal bone marrow distribution. This problem may be overcome by late imaging (after 20–24 hours). In PJI, further accumulation of labeled leukocytes is seen in the late images due to increased uptake in infected areas and reduction in background activity.[24] Labeled leukocyte scintigraphy has other important drawbacks, including its complexity, high costs, potential hazards due to the direct handling of blood products, and considerable radiation burden.[25] Fludeoxyglucose F 18 (^{18}F-FDG) PET is practically superior, because it is routinely available, provides a completed examination within 1 hour after ^{18}F-FDG administration (rather than 24 hours for labeled leukocyte imaging), and has a favorable safety profile (lack of pathogens in the final product).[25]

PRINCIPLE OF FLUDEOXYGLUCOSE F 18 POSITRON EMISSION TOMOGRAPHY IN INFECTION

Activated leukocytes use glucose as an energy source and show increased expression of glucose transporters.[23,26] In inflammatory conditions, the affinity of glucose transporters for ^{18}F-FDG is increased by various cytokines and growth factors. ^{18}F-FDG is transported into cells by glucose transporters and is phosphorylated by hexokinase enzyme to ^{18}F-FDG-6 phosphate but is not metabolized. The degree of ^{18}F-FDG uptake is related to

Table 2
Global, descriptive overview of the accuracy of different imaging modalities that may be used to diagnose periprosthetic joint infection

Imaging Modality	Sensitivity	Specificity
Radiography	Low	Low
CT	Unclear[a]	Unclear[a]
MRI	Unclear[a]	Unclear[a]
Bone scintigraphy	High	Low
Labeled leukocyte imaging	Fairly high	Fairly high
^{18}F-FDG PET	Fairly high	Fairly high

Note that accuracy may depend, among others, on diagnostic criteria used and joint site.
[a] Insufficient data.

the metabolic rate and the number of glucose transporters in leukocytes.[26] The uptake of ^{18}F-FDG reflects in vivo labeling of the existing and activated cells at the site of PJI soon after ^{18}F-FDG injection.[27] In contrast to labeled leukocyte imaging, ^{18}F-FDG uptake does not rely on leukocyte migration. Therefore, treatment with antibiotics is less likely to affect its sensitivity in delineating the PJI site.[27]

FLUDEOXYGLUCOSE F 18 POSITRON EMISSION TOMOGRAPHY PROTOCOL

Recommendations with regard to patient preparation and precautions, ^{18}F-FDG dose, and image acquisition have been outlined in detail in the European Association of Nuclear Medicine/Society of Nuclear Medicine and Molecular Imaging guideline for ^{18}F-FDG use in inflammation and infection.[28] Simultaneous PET and CT (integrated PET/CT) allows for precise allocation of ^{18}F-FDG uptake.[29] CT-based PET attenuation correction is susceptible to errors where artifacts occur, particularly in the vicinity of metal implants.[30,31] This can result in underestimation and overestimation of ^{18}F-FDG uptake.[30,31] There has been recent interest in the use of iterative metal artifact reduction of CT data, which improves PET image quality around prostheses.[30,31]

DIAGNOSTIC PERFORMANCE OF FLUDEOXYGLUCOSE F 18 POSITRON EMISSION TOMOGRAPHY

The diagnostic performance of ^{18}F-FDG PET in detecting PJI in hip and knee replacements seems sufficiently high for routine clinical application and has not proved inferior to labeled leukocyte scintigraphy.[21,22,25,27] A meta-analysis reported a pooled sensitivity of 86% (95% CI, 80% to 90%) and a pooled specificity of 93% (95% CI, 90% to 95%) for hip prostheses.[22] Another meta-analysis reported a pooled sensitivity of 70% (95% CI, 56% to 81%) and a pooled specificity of 84% (95% CI, 76% to 90%) for knee prostheses.[21] In addition, ^{18}F-FDG PET has shown useful in

patients with nonspecific clinical presentation (ie, without apparent clinical signs and symptoms, such as absence of a sinus tract).[32,33] Furthermore, it has additional value to conventional tests (including radiography, erythrocyte sedimentation rate [ESR]/C-reactive protein [CRP] testing, and joint aspiration culture and white blood cell count) in diagnosing PJI (ie, it increases accuracy).[33]

FLUDEOXYGLUCOSE F 18 POSITRON EMISSION TOMOGRAPHY EVALUATION

It is important to be aware that ^{18}F-FDG PET uptake in healing bone is normal within 3 months after surgery.[34] Differentiating between PJI and inflammation secondary due to foreign body reaction and/or aseptic loosening can be difficult. In noninfected hip prostheses, ^{18}F-FDG uptake is commonly seen around the neck[35–38] (**Figs. 1** and **2**), which may be explained by wear of components and an adverse tissue reaction.[35] Furthermore, physiologic ^{18}F-FDG uptake also may be present at the lateral and medial sides of the acetabular cup[35] (see **Fig. 2**), at the proximal portion of the femoral component,[38] and at the distal tip of the femoral component.[36] The level of physiologic ^{18}F-FDG uptake in uncemented hip prostheses is influenced by the age and probably the type of prosthesis.[35] In noninfected hip prostheses, there should be no ^{18}F-FDG uptake in the periprosthetic soft tissues, except for the soft tissue near the greater trochanter.[35] ^{18}F-FDG PET can identify soft tissue abscesses, which are not apparent on clinical examination (**Fig. 3**) and, when present, it justifies the condition of major criteria for the diagnosis of PJI.[11,12] ^{18}F-FDG uptake at the middle portion of the femoral shaft is virtually never seen in asymptomatic patients or in those with aseptic loosening and is highly suspicious for PJI (**Fig. 4**).[35,36,38,39] Most studies that have been performed to date have evaluated visual ^{18}F-FDG uptake patterns associated with aseptic loosening or PJI. There is no accepted standardized uptake value (SUV) threshold to diagnose PJI. More importantly, the intensity of

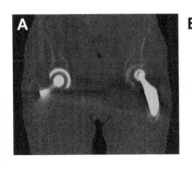
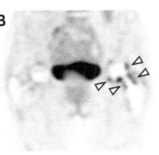

Fig. 1. Nonspecific ^{18}F-FDG uptake in a 66-year-old woman with bilateral asymptomatic total hip prostheses. This patient underwent ^{18}F-FDG PET to evaluate a lung lesion. Coronal PET image (*B*) shows nonspecific ^{18}F-FDG uptake around the neck of the left hip prosthesis (*arrowheads*), with corresponding CT image (*A*).

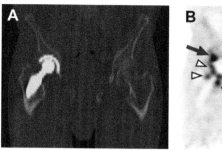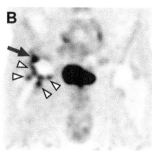

Fig. 2. Nonspecific ^{18}F-FDG uptake in a 70-year-old man with asymptomatic right total hip prosthesis. This patient underwent ^{18}F-FDG PET to identify the cause of fever of unknown origin. Coronal PET image (*B*) shows nonspecific ^{18}F-FDG uptake around the neck (*arrowheads*) and nonspecific ^{18}F-FDG uptake at lateral side of the acetabular cup (*arrow*), with corresponding CT image (*A*).

^{18}F-FDG uptake is less important than the location of increased ^{18}F-FDG uptake to diagnose PJI.[40] Hip prostheses, which show aseptic loosening, can be accompanied by an intense inflammatory response involving large numbers of leukocytes[41] and, as a result, demonstrate intense ^{18}F-FDG uptake, with SUVs as high as 7.[40] Therefore, using increased ^{18}F-FDG uptake as the sole criterion to diagnose PJI in hip prostheses results in false-positive results.[40] The pattern of ^{18}F-FDG uptake around noninfected knee prostheses has been less well documented than that of hip prostheses. Nonspecific synovial ^{18}F-FDG uptake in knee prostheses has been reported by several studies[42–45] (**Fig. 5**). On the other hand, ^{18}F-FDG uptake at the bone-prosthesis interface of the

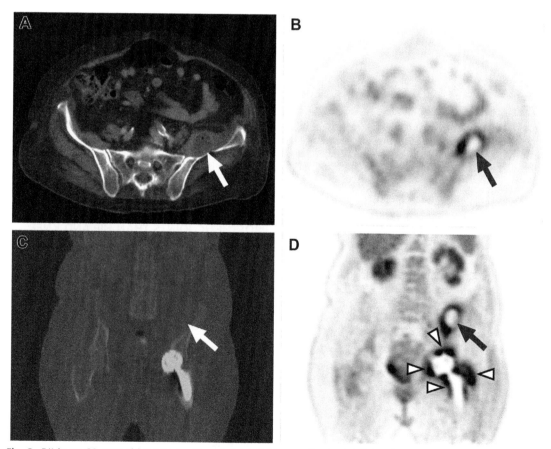

Fig. 3. PJI in an 80-year-old woman with painful left hip prosthesis. Axial (*A, B*) and coronal (*C, D*) CT and PET images are displayed. There is a fluid collection in the left iliacus (*arrows* [*A, C*]) muscle, which shows peripheral ^{18}F-FDG uptake and no central ^{18}F-FDG uptake (*arrows* [*B, D*]), compatible with an abscess. This abscess was not suspected clinically and extended caudally to the left hip joint. In addition, there is ^{18}F-FDG uptake at the bone-prosthesis interface around the acetabular cup and at the proximal femoral stem (*arrowheads* [*D*]).

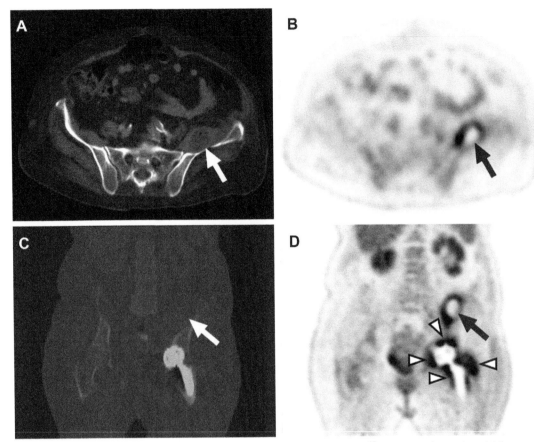

Fig. 4. PJI in a patient with bilateral prosthesis. Coronal PET image reveals ^{18}F-FDG uptake at the middle portion of the femoral shaft at the bone-prosthesis interface (*arrow*), which is highly suspicious for PJI. PJI was confirmed by further assessment. (*From* Saboury B, Ziai P, Parsons M, et al. Promising Roles of PET in Management of Arthroplasty-Associated Infection. PET Clin 2012; 7:139-50; with permission.)

femoral or tibial component has been consistently reported as diagnostic criterion for PJI in knee prostheses[21] (**Fig. 6**). The influence of ^{18}F-FDG uptake, however, at specific bone-prosthesis locations on diagnostic performance has not been reported yet, to the authors' knowledge. **Table 3** summarizes areas of nonspecific ^{18}F-FDG uptake and criteria for PJI in hip and knee prostheses, based on available evidence.

ROLE OF FLUDEOXYGLUCOSE F 18 POSITRON EMISSION TOMOGRAPHY IN OTHER PROSTHETIC JOINTS THAN HIP AND KNEE

The number of shoulder replacements is growing faster than ever.[46] The occurrence rate of PJI after total shoulder replacement is approximately 1% to 3.9% and can be even higher in reversed designs due to an increase in dead space and hematoma formation.[47] Of all revision shoulder operations,

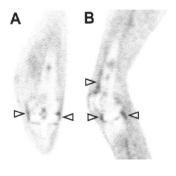
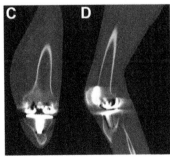

Fig. 5. Nonspecific synovial ^{18}F-FDG uptake in an asymptomatic knee prosthesis of a 70-year-old man, as shown on coronal (*A*) and sagittal (*B*) PET images (*arrowheads*), with corresponding CT images (*C, D*).

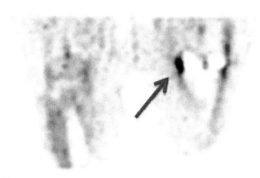

Fig. 6. PJI in a patient with a left knee prosthesis. Coronal PET image demonstrates a focus of intense ^{18}F-FDG uptake in the medial aspect of femoral component at the bone-prosthesis interface (*arrow*). Operative findings and histopathology confirmed the presence of infection. (*From* Saboury B, Ziai P, Parsons M, et al. Promising Roles of PET in Management of Arthroplasty-Associated Infection. PET Clin 2012; 7:139-50; with permission.)

12% are due to PJI.[47] Because the number of patients who undergo shoulder arthroplasty is growing fast,[46,47] it can be anticipated that the number of patients with PJI also will increase. The value of ^{18}F-FDG PET in evaluating shoulder PJI, however, has not yet been extensively investigated. The results of a recent study suggested that ^{18}F-FDG PET has poor diagnostic accuracy in diagnosing low-grade PJI of the shoulder.[48] In addition, the performance and place of ^{18}F-FDG

PET in the diagnostic decision tree of suspected PJI in other less common arthroplasty sites, such as the elbow and ankle, also remains to be investigated. The potential of ^{18}F-FDG PET in evaluating elbow prosthesis already has been demonstrated,[49] but diagnostic accuracy data are not available yet.

FUTURE PERSPECTIVES

Although diagnostic performance of ^{18}F-FDG PET in detecting hip and knee PJI seems sufficiently high for clinical use, results from several individual studies were heterogeneous.[21,22] Importantly, the definition of PJI has evolved over the years with the most recent updated evidence-based and validated definition for PJI published in 2018.[12] Most ^{18}F-FDG PET studies performed so far, however, used various other/older definitions of PJI, which may have been an important source of heterogeneity. Standardization of ^{18}F-FDG PET acquisition protocols, diagnostic criteria, and reference standard is required to further explore potential causes of heterogeneity (including type and age of prosthesis) and to further validate this method, preferably by multicenter studies. Large prospective studies comparing the diagnostic performance of ^{18}F-FDG PET and labeled leukocyte imaging for PJI are anticipated.[14] Simultaneous PET and MRI (integrated PET/MRI) has high potential to improve the noninvasive diagnosis of PJI in 1 single examination, because it combines the functional information gathered from PET and the excellent anatomic detail and soft tissue contrast from MRI.[50]

SUMMARY

Diagnosing PJI can be a challenge, especially for chronic and low-grade infections. The diagnostic performance of ^{18}F-FDG PET in detecting PJI in hip and knee replacements seems sufficiently high for routine clinical application and adds to conventional tests. Location rather than intensity of ^{18}F-FDG uptake is critical in diagnosing hip and knee PJI. ^{18}F-FDG uptake at the middle portion of the femoral component and ^{18}F-FDG uptake at the bone-prosthesis interface can be considered positive criteria for PJI in hip and knee prostheses, respectively. The role of ^{18}F-FDG PET in other prosthetic joints remains to be investigated.

DISCLOSURE

All authors have no disclosures to declare.

Table 3
Areas of nonspecific fludeoxyglucose F 18 uptake and criteria for periprosthetic joint infection in hip and knee prostheses, based on available evidence

	Areas of Nonspecific Fludeoxyglucose F 18 Uptake	Criteria for Periprosthetic Joint Infection
Hip	• Around the neck of the prosthesis • Lateral and medial sides of the acetabular cup • Proximal portion of the femoral component • Distal portion of the femoral component	• ^{18}F-FDG uptake at the middle portion of the femoral component
Knee	• Synovium	• ^{18}F-FDG uptake at the bone-prosthesis interface

REFERENCES

1. Maradit Kremers H, Larson DR, Crowson CS, et al. Prevalence of total hip and knee replacement in the United States. J Bone Joint Surg Am 2015;97: 1386–97.
2. Lam V, Teutsch S, Fielding J. Hip and knee replacements: a neglected potential savings opportunity. JAMA 2018;319:977–8.
3. van der Wees PJ, Wammes JJ, Akkermans RP, et al. Patient-reported health outcomes after total hip and knee surgery in a Dutch University Hospital Setting: results of twenty years clinical registry. BMC Musculoskelet Disord 2017;18:97.
4. Labek G, Thaler M, Janda W, et al. Revision rates after total joint replacement: cumulative results from worldwide joint register datasets. J Bone Joint Surg Br 2011;93:293–7.
5. Kapadia BH, Berg RA, Daley JA, et al. Periprosthetic joint infection. Lancet 2016;387:386–94.
6. Alp E, Cevahir F, Ersoy S, et al. Incidence and economic burden of prosthetic joint infections in a university hospital: a report from a middle-income country. J Infect Public Health 2016;9:494–8.
7. Kurtz SM, Lau E, Watson H, et al. Economic burden of periprosthetic joint infection in the United States. J Arthroplasty 2012;27(8 Suppl):61–5.
8. Charette RS, Melnic CM. Two-stage revision arthroplasty for the treatment of prosthetic joint infection. Curr Rev Musculoskelet Med 2018;11:332–40.
9. Tande AJ, Patel R. Prosthetic joint infection. Clin Microbiol Rev 2014;27:302–45.
10. Gbejuade HO, Lovering AM, Webb JC. The role of microbial biofilms in prosthetic joint infections. Acta Orthop 2015;86:147–58.
11. Amanatullah D, Dennis D, Oltra EG, et al. Hip and knee section, diagnosis, definitions: proceedings of International Consensus on Orthopedic Infections. J Arthroplasty 2019;34:S329–37.
12. Parvizi J, Tan TL, Goswami K, et al. The 2018 definition of periprosthetic hip and knee infection: an evidence-based and validated criteria. J Arthroplasty 2018;33:1309–14.
13. Ali F, Wilkinson JM, Cooper JR, et al. Accuracy of joint aspiration for the preoperative diagnosis of infection in total hip arthroplasty. J Arthroplasty 2006;21:221–6.
14. Signore A, Sconfienza LM, Borens O, et al. Consensus document for the diagnosis of prosthetic joint infections: a joint paper by the EANM, EBJIS, and ESR (with ESCMID endorsement). Eur J Nucl Med Mol Imaging 2019;46:971–88.
15. Li C, Renz N, Trampuz A. Management of periprosthetic joint infection. Hip Pelvis 2018;30:138–46.
16. Cyteval C, Hamm V, Sarrabère MP, et al. Painful infection at the site of hip prosthesis: CT imaging. Radiology 2002;224:477–83.
17. Fritz J, Lurie B, Miller TT, et al. MR imaging of hip arthroplasty implants. Radiographics 2014;34: E106–32.
18. Fritz J, Lurie B, Potter HG. MR imaging of knee arthroplasty implants. Radiographics 2015;35: 1483–501.
19. Koff MF, Burge AJ, Koch KM, et al. Imaging near orthopedic hardware. J Magn Reson Imaging 2017; 46:24–39.
20. Grant FD, Fahey FH, Packard AB, et al. Skeletal PET with 18F-fluoride: applying new technology to an old tracer. J Nucl Med 2008;49:68–78.
21. Verberne SJ, Sonnega RJ, Temmerman OP, et al. What is the accuracy of nuclear imaging in the assessment of periprosthetic knee infection? A meta-analysis. Clin Orthop Relat Res 2017;475: 1395–410.
22. Verberne SJ, Raijmakers PG, Temmerman OP. The accuracy of imaging techniques in the assessment of periprosthetic hip infection: a systematic review and meta-analysis. J Bone Joint Surg Am 2016;98: 1638–45.
23. Glaudemans AW, Galli F, Pacilio M, et al. Leukocyte and bacteria imaging in prosthetic joint infection. Eur Cell Mater 2013;25:61–77.
24. Signore A, Jamar F, Israel O, et al. Clinical indications, image acquisition and data interpretation for white blood cells and anti-granulocyte monoclonal antibody scintigraphy: an EANM procedural guideline. Eur J Nucl Med Mol Imaging 2018;45:1816–31.
25. Kwee TC, Basu S, Alavi A. The ongoing misperception that labeled leukocyte imaging is superior to 18F-FDG PET for diagnosing prosthetic joint infection. J Nucl Med 2017;58:182.
26. Love C, Tomas MB, Tronco GG, et al. FDG PET of infection and inflammation. Radiographics 2005;25: 1357–68.
27. Basu S, Kwee TC, Saboury B, et al. FDG PET for diagnosing infection in hip and knee prostheses: prospective study in 221 prostheses and subgroup comparison with combined (111)In-labeled leukocyte/(99m)Tc-sulfur colloid bone marrow imaging in 88 prostheses. Clin Nucl Med 2014;39: 609–15.
28. Jamar F, Buscombe J, Chiti A, et al. EANM/SNMMI guideline for 18F-FDG use in inflammation and infection. J Nucl Med 2013;54:647–58.
29. von Schulthess GK, Steinert HC, Hany TF. Integrated PET/CT: current applications and future directions. Radiology 2006;238:405–22.
30. van der Vos CS, Arens AIJ, Hamill JJ, et al. Metal artifact reduction of CT scans to improve PET/CT. J Nucl Med 2017;58:1867–72.
31. Schabel C, Gatidis S, Bongers M, et al. Improving CT-based PET attenuation correction in the vicinity of metal implants by an iterative metal artifact reduction algorithm of CT data and its comparison to

dual-energy-based strategies: a phantom study. Invest Radiol 2017;52:61–5.

32. Zajonz D, Zieme A, Prietzel T, et al. Periprosthetic joint infections in modular endoprostheses of the lower extremities: a retrospective observational study in 101 patients. Patient Saf Surg 2016;10:6.

33. Kwee RM, Broos WA, Brans B, et al. Added value of 18F-FDG PET/CT in diagnosing infected hip prosthesis. Acta Radiol 2018;59:569–76.

34. Zhuang H, Sam JW, Chacko TK, et al. Rapid normalization of osseous FDG uptake following traumatic or surgical fractures. Eur J Nucl Med Mol Imaging 2003;30:1096–103.

35. Gelderman SJ, Jutte PC, Boellaard R, et al. 18F-FDG-PET uptake in non-infected total hip prostheses. Acta Orthop 2018;89:634–9.

36. Zhuang H, Chacko TK, Hickeson M, et al. Persistent non-specific FDG uptake on PET imaging following hip arthroplasty. Eur J Nucl Med Mol Imaging 2002;29:1328–33.

37. Vanquickenborne B, Maes A, Nuyts J, et al. The value of (18)FDG-PET for the detection of infected hip prosthesis. Eur J Nucl Med Mol Imaging 2003; 30(5):705–15.

38. Aydin A, Yu JQ, Zhuang H, et al. Patterns of 18F-FDG PET images in patients with uncomplicated total hip arthroplasty. Hell J Nucl Med 2015;18:93–6.

39. Verberne SJ, Temmerman OPP, Vuong BH, et al. Fluorodeoxyglucose positron emission tomography imaging for diagnosing periprosthetic hip infection: the importance of diagnostic criteria. Int Orthop 2018; 42:2025–34.

40. Chacko TK, Zhuang H, Stevenson K, et al. The importance of the location of fluorodeoxyglucose uptake in periprosthetic infection in painful hip prostheses. Nucl Med Commun 2002;23:851–5.

41. Palestro CJ. Radionuclide imaging of musculoskeletal infection: a review. J Nucl Med 2016;57: 1406–12.

42. Love C, Marwin SE, Tomas MB, et al. Diagnosing infection in the failed joint replacement: a comparison of coincidence detection 18F-FDG and 111In-labeled leukocyte/99mTc-sulfur colloid marrow imaging. J Nucl Med 2004;45:1864–71.

43. Delank KS, Schmidt M, Michael JW, et al. The implications of 18F-FDG PET for the diagnosis of endoprosthetic loosening and infection in hip and knee arthroplasty: results from a prospective, blinded study. BMC Musculoskelet Disord 2006;7:20.

44. Van Acker F, Nuyts J, Maes A, et al. FDG-PET, 99mtc-HMPAO white blood cell SPET and bone scintigraphy in the evaluation of painful total knee arthroplasties. Eur J Nucl Med 2001;28:1496–504.

45. Mayer-Wagner S, Mayer W, Maegerlein S, et al. Use of 18F-FDG-PET in the diagnosis of endoprosthetic loosening of knee and hip implants. Arch Orthop Trauma Surg 2010;130:1231–8.

46. Kim SH, Wise BL, Zhang Y, et al. Increasing incidence of shoulder arthroplasty in the United States. J Bone Joint Surg Am 2011;93:2249–54.

47. Pinder EM, Ong JC, Bale RS, et al. Ten questions on prosthetic shoulder infection. Shoulder Elbow 2016; 8:151–7.

48. Falstie-Jensen T, Daugaard H, Søballe K, et al, ROSA Study Group. Labeled white blood cell/bone marrow single-photon emission computed tomography with computed tomography fails in diagnosing chronic periprosthetic shoulder joint infection. J Shoulder Elbow Surg 2019;28:1040–8.

49. Balasubramanian Harisankar Natrajan C, Mittal BR, Bhattacharya A, et al. Interesting image. Aseptic loosening of elbow prostheses diagnosed on F-18 FDG PET/CT. Clin Nucl Med 2010;35:886–7.

50. Ehman EC, Johnson GB, Villanueva-Meyer JE, et al. PET/MRI: where might it replace PET/CT? J Magn Reson Imaging 2017;46:1247–62.

PET Scan with Fludeoxyglucose/ Computed Tomography in Low-Grade Vascular Inflammation

Aarthi S. Reddy, BS, Domingo E. Uceda, BS, Mina Al Najafi, MD,
Amit K. Dey, MD, Nehal N. Mehta, MD, MSCE*

KEYWORDS

- Fluorodeoxyglucose-positron emission tomography/computed tomography • Inflammation
- Vascular disease

KEY POINTS

- Fluorodeoxyglucose-PET/computed tomography combines the high sensitivity of PET with the excellent spatial resolution provided by computed tomography, making it a potentially powerful tool for capturing and quantifying early vascular diseases.
- Patients with chronic inflammatory states have an increased risk of cardiovascular events as well as increased vascular fluorodeoxyglucose uptake compared with healthy controls.
- Fluorodeoxyglucose-PET/computed tomography can be used as a reliable tool to assess low-grade vascular inflammation including responses to treatment in chronic inflammatory disease states.

INTRODUCTION

Cardiovascular disease (CVD), including atherosclerosis, is the leading cause of death worldwide and therefore significant efforts to capture early subclinical vascular disease have been made in the past decade. In this context, fluorodeoxyglucose PET/computed tomography (FDG PET/CT) uses a radiolabeled glucose analogue taken up by cells in the vessel wall in direct proportion to their metabolic activity. FDG PET/CT combines the high sensitivity of PET for the detection of inflammation using the spatial resolution and morphologic information provided by CT.[1] This review covers how FDG PET/CT has been used to detect subclinical vascular disease in various inflammatory states.

Low-Grade Vascular Inflammation in Chronic Inflammatory States

Chronic inflammatory diseases are associated with a high incidence of CV events.[2] Inflammation and lipid dysfunction associates with initiation and progression of atherosclerosis. Systemic inflammatory biomarkers, such as high-sensitivity C-reactive protein, have been associated with atherosclerotic disease and future CV events.[3] Moreover, inflammatory cells, such as circulating monocytes, have been useful in detecting plaque vulnerability[4] and distinct monocyte subpopulations are significantly associated with subclinical atherosclerosis.[5] Chronic inflammatory diseases, including psoriasis, rheumatoid arthritis (RA), systemic lupus erythematosus, and persons living

Funding: None.
Section of Inflammation and Cardiometabolic Diseases, National Heart, Lung and Blood Institute, Clinical Research Center, 10 Center Drive, Room 5-5140, Bethesda, MD 20892, USA
* Corresponding author.
E-mail address: nehal.mehta@nih.gov

PET Clin 15 (2020) 207–213
https://doi.org/10.1016/j.cpet.2019.11.009
1556-8598/20/Published by Elsevier Inc.

with human immunodeficiency virus (HIV), have all been independently associated with increased risk of CV disease.[6] Compared with age- and gender-matched controls, these patients have heightened macrophage activity and inflammatory cytokines including tumor necrosis factor (TNF)-α IL-6, IL-1 and IL-17A, all of which have been linked to key pathways contributing to atherogenesis. Because of this, individuals with chronic inflammatory states are at higher risk for inflammatory driven CV disease compared with their healthy counterparts.[2,6] In these patients there is an unmet need to detect subclinical vascular disease before CV events occur.

Vascular Uptake of Fludeoxyglucose by PET/Computed Tomography

Early atherosclerotic lesions have increased presence of myeloid-derived immune cells; lesion progression is accelerated by their secreted products and subsequent chemotaxis. First, a lesion in the blood vessel begins with a fatty streak, an accumulation of lipids and macrophages beneath the endothelium. Next asymmetric, focal thickening of the intima occurs, consisting of foam cells, proinflammatory macrophages, oxidized lipoproteins, and extracellular lipid droplets, all surrounded by fibrous cap consisting of smooth muscle cells and a collagen-rich matrix.[7,8] Atherosclerotic plaques differ in risk of rupture based on several features. High-risk plaques have a thin fibrous cap, a lipid necrotic core, microcalcifications, neovascularization, and an abundance of activated immune cells.[8] Plaque rupture leads to intraluminal thrombus formation via exposure of the thrombogenic core to circulating platelets and clotting factors. Notably, a potent driver for plaque destabilization and subsequent CV events is inflammation. ^{18}F-FDG is a radiolabeled glucose analogue that is taken up by glucose transporters and phosphorylated by hexokinase, the enzyme responsible for the first step in glycolysis. Normally, glucose's 2-hydroxyl group is then used for further glycolysis; however, because ^{18}F-FDG lacks this 2-hydroxy group, it cannot be further processed nor can it leave the cell before radioactive decay. ^{18}F-FDG accumulation at sites of acute and chronic inflammation is primarily owing to an overexpression of glucose transporters as well as hexokinase in active inflammatory cells.[9] Furthermore, when compared with resting macrophages, activated macrophages have a dramatically increased level of hexokinase activity.[10] Vascular FDG uptake in subclinical atherosclerosis, a chronic low-grade inflammatory disease, has long been documented through PET imaging

in major vessels throughout the body, usually the aorta, carotids, and most recently the coronary arteries.[11] FDG PET uptake was first incidentally noted in the vascular wall of large arteries, during an oncologic-indicated examination, and found that FDG vascular uptake correlated with CV risk factors.[12] Validation of FDG PET as a marker of the inflammation in an atherosclerotic plaque originated from in vitro histology studies, including immunostaining for macrophages in endarterectomy samples from carotid plaques.[13,14] There is an upregulation of CD68, a recognized marker of macrophages, in lesions with increased FDG uptake. Subsequent clinical studies of FDG PET/CT showed that CT-derived vascular calcification and PET metabolic activity in fact were detecting potentially different stages of plaque development.[15] Additionally, high-risk plaque morphology by CT corresponded with the inflammation burden detected by FDG PET.[16]

Inflammatory vascular conditions also show extensive FDG PET uptake in blood vessel walls. Most notable is central and peripheral vasculitis, which generally affects the medium to large vessels preferentially. Additionally, FDG PET uptake occurs in vascular graft-related infection, intravascular thrombosis, vascular tumors, fistulas and aneurysms.[17] Symptomatic aortic aneurysms have increased FDG uptake and this potentially may associate with rupture risk.[18] FDG PET/CT also has a role in detecting and quantifying aortitis of infectious and noninfectious etiologies. Most notably, FDG PET/CT has a very high sensitivity and specificity in the diagnosis of large vessel vasculitis, such as Takayasu arteritis and giant cell arteritis, which typically affect the large arteries of the body such as the aorta and its major branches. FDG uptake in large vessel vasculitis is characteristically lineal diffuse uptake, differentiated from low-grade patchy uptake seen in atherosclerotic vessels, and is in increased in patients with large vessel vasculitis compared with controls.[19] Furthermore, although rare, FDG PET/CT can be useful in the evaluation of indolent primary aortic malignancies, most commonly sarcomas, and embolic spread, distant metastasis, or extension into adjacent arteries.[18]

PET with Fludeoxyglucose/Computed Tomography and the Association with Vascular Disease

The Cardiovascular Committee of the European Association of Nuclear Medicine recently recommended standardized protocols for imaging and interpretation of atherosclerosis imaging via FDG PET/CT; however, the lack of conclusive evidence limits these recommendations.[20] Despite this, multiple prospective studies have shown relationships of increased aortic vascular inflammation in atherosclerosis by FDG PET/CT with higher incidence of CVD, including myocardial infarction, heart failure, and peripheral claudication. FDG PET has been used to image vascular uptake in the aorta, carotid arteries, and coronary arteries.[21]

Inflammatory disease states have been associated with a higher incidence of vascular disease compared with age- and gender-matched controls.[21] In chronic low-grade inflammatory states such as psoriasis, RA, HIV, and systemic lupus erythematosus, vascular FDG uptake is higher compared with controls (**Fig. 1**).[21,22-25] In a case-control study, increased vascular FDG uptake consistent with early vascular disease was observed in psoriasis patients compared with controls.[26] Also, psoriasis severity and markers of neutrophil activation associated with vascular inflammation assessed as the target-to-background ratio (TBR) in the aorta (maximal standardized uptake value in the artery to mean standardized uptake value in the vein) beyond traditional CV risk factors.[27] Additionally, in 91 patients with RA without CVD, increased FDG uptake was associated with RA disease activity.[24] Finally, individuals with systemic lupus erythematosus and HIV had increased vascular inflammation by FDG PET/CT compared with healthy controls.[22,25] These studies demonstrate the ability of FDG PET/CT to be used as a tool in detecting aortic vascular inflammation in patients with inflammatory disease without clinical CVD.

FDG PET is also used to assess carotid disease. Rudd et. all first reported that in 8 patients with symptomatic carotid disease there was increased FDG accumulation in macrophage-dense regions of carotid artery plaques compared with asymptomatic plaques, with no uptake in normal arteries.[13] Later, increased ipsilateral FDG PET uptake as measured by maximal standardized uptake value ratios in atherosclerotic carotid lesions was associated with a close time interval to events such as stroke or transient ischemic attack when compared with those with solely chronic obstructive stenosis,[28] suggesting that FDG PET/CT may be used to tailor stroke prevention strategies.[29]

Recently, FDG uptake in the aorta has been associated with coronary plaque characteristics by coronary CT angiography (CCTA), providing further evidence for FDG/PET in capturing subclinical atherosclerosis.[30] High vascular FDG uptake was associated with high-risk plaque detected by CCTA in psoriasis and HIV (**Fig. 2**).[30,31] Finally, increased FDG PET uptake has been shown to be associated with culprit coronary lesions in the left main coronary artery in patients presenting with acute coronary syndromes[11]; however, spatial resolution of PET precludes future use for coronary imaging at this time.

PET with Fludeoxyglucose/Computed Tomography and Response to Treatment

Vascular FDG uptake allows for detection of changes in aortic vascular inflammation in response to classical coronary artery disease interventions. Primary prevention of coronary artery

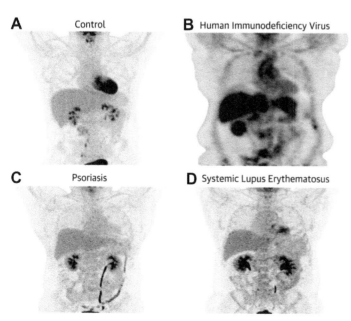

A Control
B Human Immunodeficiency Virus
C Psoriasis
D Systemic Lupus Erythematosus

Fig. 1. Aortic vascular FDG uptake in various chronically inflamed human models. Representative ^{18}F-FDG PET/CT imaging of the aorta in a healthy control (A), patient with HIV (B), psoriasis (C), and systemic lupus erythematosus (D).

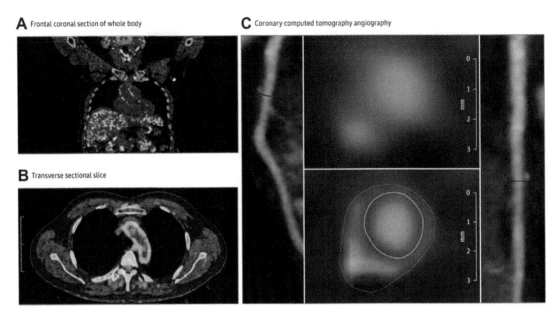

A Frontal coronal section of whole body

B Transverse sectional slice

C Coronary computed tomography angiography

Fig. 2. Aortic vascular uptake of FDG by PET/CT scan and coronary artery disease characterization by CCTA. Frontal coronal section of whole body FDG PET/CT scan with increased uptake of FDG throughout the body, specifically in the aortic wall, in a patient with psoriasis (*A*). Transverse sectional slice from FDG PET/CT that shows increased vascular FDG uptake in the aortic wall (*green*) in a patient with psoriasis (*B*). Reconstructed images from CCTA. Left anterior descending coronary artery (*left*) depicts noncalcified burden of the coronary artery and transverse section of left anterior descending coronary artery (*right*). The planar reconstruction (*middle*) demonstrates low-attenuation lipid-rich high-risk plaque (*green* and *red*).

disease is centered on risk factor control and improvements in lifestyle, which have been shown to modify vascular inflammation as detected by FDG PET/CT. In a study assessing 60 adults who underwent both atherogenic risk factor assessment and FDG PET/CT at baseline and again after 17 months of follow-up after intense lifestyle modification, changes in CV risk factors, including diastolic blood pressure, total cholesterol, and low-density lipoprotein, as well as increase in high-density lipoprotein, were associated with a decreased vascular inflammation by FDG PET/CT.[32]

Currently, statins are commonly used for maintaining and preventing CVD. HMG-CoA reductase or statins have been shown to decrease vascular uptake of FDG and this decrease is later mirrored by a concordant reduction in CVD events. A prior study demonstrated that intense statin therapy led to a reduction in atherosclerotic inflammation as measured by FDG PET/CT. Eighty-three adults with known atherosclerotic disease not on high-intensity statin therapy were serially imaged with FDG PET/CT at baseline, 4, and 12 weeks follow-up after randomization to low- or high-dose statin therapy. Vascular inflammation as assessed by FDG PET-CT TBR was significantly reduced in the high-dose statin group (atorvastatin 80 mg) compared with the low-dose statin group

(atorvastatin 10 mg) [change in TBR from baseline to 4 weeks 80 mg: 7.6 (range, 2.6–12.3) vs 10 mg: 2.0 (range, −3.1 to 6.8) and change in TBR from baseline to 12 weeks 80 mg: 6.7 (range, 1.8–11.3) versus 10 mg: −0.1 (range, −5.6 to 5.1)].[33]

Novel emerging medications and their influence on vascular inflammation may also be assessed by FDG PET/CT to support or refute clinical trials of emerging drugs. The p38 map kinase inhibitors notably were not associated with decreased vascular FDG uptake. Later, a follow-up events study failed to demonstrate that p38 map kinase inhibition had any impact on CVD events. Therefore, small-scale FDG PET/CT imaging trials may be useful in identifying strategies that may have promise to reduce CV events in larger endpoint trials. The impact of primary disease therapy on vascular inflammation has been assessed by FDG PET. Notably, anti–TNF-α, as well as anti-IL12/23, anti-IL17, and anti-IL-1β therapies are all indicated in the treatment of inflammatory skin and joint diseases. Small observational preliminary findings implied that initiating a biologic treatment, such as anti-TNF, precedes a decrease in vascular inflammation by arterial FDG uptake[23,34]; however, randomized controlled trials showed no effect of anti-TNF therapy at follow-up. The Vascular Inflammation in Psoriasis trial aimed to understand the impact of anticytokine treatments on vascular disease. Through a series of randomized, placebo-controlled trials, anti-TNF therapy was found to have no impact on vascular inflammation by FDG PET compared with a placebo.[35] In contrast, anti-IL12/23 therapy resulted in an initial transient reduction in aortic vascular inflammation.[36] Moreover, antiretroviral therapies that were studied using FDG PET have shown no effect on vascular inflammation.[37]

Limitations

FDG PET/CT is useful in detecting vascular inflammation, but it also has certain clinical and analytical limitations. Clinical factors such as prescan glucose levels and high body mass index (BMI) can influence FDG uptake values. As prescan glucose levels increase, there is a decrease in FDG uptake owing to the competition between glucose and FDG; therefore prescan glucose levels of greater than 200 mg/dL should be avoided to improve tracer uptake. Those with an increased BMI additionally have worse image quality compared with those with normal BMI owing to scatter. These limitations can be somewhat overcome by increasing the injected dose of radiotracer or increasing the acquisition time of scan; however, these strategies have led to little improvement.[38] Additionally, imaging protocols such as patient preparation and timing of imaging are all potential patient factors that can impact the measured FDG uptake. Protocols often differ in scan acquisition times, and can vary from 1 to 3 hours; however, fortunately numerous studies have shown that a circulation time of more than 2 hours gives a higher TBR.[39] Furthermore, background variability is also a limitation. Specifically, background blood activity is often normalized when quantifying TBR; however, because of fundamental differences in blood pool activity, TBR values may be influenced. Moreover, the choice of background tissue also affects TBR uptake values. Last, the spatial resolution of PET imaging can be difficult when attempting to capture uptake in small structures owing to the partial volume effect; however, coupling PET with CT scans has substantially overcome this limitation. In attempts to offer a higher quality of information, PET scanners have undergone notable improvements. One such advancement is the time of flight PET scanner. The current generation time of flight PET scanners offer a higher resolution and have the ability to operate in a 3-dimensional mode.[40]

Furthermore, the time of flight PET scanner can be used with patients who have higher BMIs, allowing PET CT scans to accommodate for many more patients.[8] Although there are many factors that can introduce variation in FDG uptake in the vessel, many can be controlled for; however, careful analysis of results is required.

Future Directions

FDG PET/CT scans overall show promise in detecting subclinical vascular inflammation and changes in vascular inflammation may indicate disease progression or improvement with interventions. Notably, FDG PET/CT scans have been used in detecting culprit coronary lesions; however, the associated technical limitations, including high myocardial FDG uptake, cardiac motion, and the small size of plaque, make its application difficult. There are promising methods to overcome high myocardial FDG uptake that can be accomplished by have patients trial a high-fat, low-carbohydrate diet before imaging[41] and thus its role in coronary inflammation has yet to be elucidated.

DISCLOSURES

NNM is a full-time US government employee and has served as a consultant for Amgen, Eli Lilly, and Leo Pharma, receiving grants/other payments; as a principal investigator and/or investigator for AbbVie, Celgene, Janssen Pharmaceuticals, and Novartis, receiving grants and/or research funding; and as a principal investigator for the National Institutes of Health, receiving grants and/or research funding. DEU is funded by the NIH Medical Research Scholars Program, a public–private partnership supported jointly by the NIH and generous contributions to the Foundation for the NIH from the Doris Duke Charitable Foundation (DDCF Grant # 2014194), Genentech, Elsevier, and other private donors. All other authors have no conflict of interest.

REFERENCES

1. Chaturvedi A, Dey AK, Joshi AA, et al. Vascular inflammation imaging in psoriasis. Curr Cardiovasc Imaging Rep 2017;10(2):4.
2. Deeks SG, Tracy R, Douek DC. Systemic effects of inflammation on health during chronic HIV infection. Immunity 2013;39(4):633–45.
3. Ridker PM, Cushman M, Stampfer MJ, et al. Inflammation, aspirin, and the risk of cardiovascular disease in apparently healthy men. N Engl J Med 1997;336(14):973–9.
4. Gordon S, Taylor PR. Monocyte and macrophage heterogeneity. Nat Rev Immunol 2005;5(12):953–64.

5. Rogacev KS, Ulrich C, Blomer L, et al. Monocyte heterogeneity in obesity and subclinical atherosclerosis. Eur Heart J 2010;31(3):369–76.

6. Boehncke WH. Systemic inflammation and cardiovascular comorbidity in psoriasis patients: causes and consequences. Front Immunol 2018;9(579):579.

7. Bural GG, Torigian DA, Chamroonrat W, et al. Quantitative assessment of the atherosclerotic burden of the aorta by combined FDG-PET and CT image analysis: a new concept. Nucl Med Biol 2006;33(8):1037–43.

8. Joseph P, Tawakol A. Imaging atherosclerosis with positron emission tomography. Eur Heart J 2016;37(39):2974–80.

9. Chrapko BE, Chrapko M, Nocun A, et al. Role of 18F-FDG PET/CT in the diagnosis of inflammatory and infectious vascular disease. Nucl Med Rev Cent East Eur 2016;19(1):28–36.

10. Rudd JH, Narula J, Strauss HW, et al. Imaging atherosclerotic plaque inflammation by fluorodeoxyglucose with positron emission tomography: ready for prime time? J Am Coll Cardiol 2010;55(23):2527–35.

11. Rogers IS, Nasir K, Figueroa AL, et al. Feasibility of FDG imaging of the coronary arteries: comparison between acute coronary syndrome and stable angina. JACC Cardiovasc Imaging 2010;3(4):388–97.

12. Yun M, Jang S, Cucchiara A, et al. 18F FDG uptake in the large arteries: a correlation study with the atherogenic risk factors. Semin Nucl Med 2002;32(1):70–6.

13. Rudd JH, Warburton EA, Fryer TD, et al. Imaging atherosclerotic plaque inflammation with [18F]-fluorodeoxyglucose positron emission tomography. Circulation 2002;105(23):2708–11.

14. Graebe M, Pedersen SF, Borgwardt L, et al. Molecular pathology in vulnerable carotid plaques: correlation with [18]-fluorodeoxyglucose positron emission tomography (FDG-PET). Eur J Vasc Endovasc Surg 2009;37(6):714–21.

15. Menezes LJ, Kotze CW, Agu O, et al. Investigating vulnerable atheroma using combined (18)F-FDG PET/CT angiography of carotid plaque with immunohistochemical validation. J Nucl Med 2011;52(11):1698–703.

16. Figueroa AL, Subramanian SS, Cury RC, et al. Distribution of inflammation within carotid atherosclerotic plaques with high-risk morphological features: a comparison between positron emission tomography activity, plaque morphology, and histopathology. Circ Cardiovasc Imaging 2012;5(1):69–77.

17. Zhuang H, Codreanu I. Growing applications of FDG PET-CT imaging in non-oncologic conditions. J Biomed Res 2015;29(3):189–202.

18. Kim J, Song HC. Role of PET/CT in the evaluation of aortic disease. Chonnam Med J 2018;54(3):143–52.

19. Lawal I, Sathekge M. F-18 FDG PET/CT imaging of cardiac and vascular inflammation and infection. Br Med Bull 2016;120(1):55–74.

20. Bucerius J, Hyafil F, Verberne HJ, et al. Position paper of the cardiovascular committee of the European association of nuclear medicine (EANM) on PET imaging of atherosclerosis. Eur J Nucl Med Mol Imaging 2016;43(4):780–92.

21. Teague HL, Ahlman MA, Alavi A, et al. Unraveling vascular inflammation: from immunology to imaging. J Am Coll Cardiol 2017;70(11):1403–12.

22. Carlucci PM, Purmalek MM, Dey AK, et al. Neutrophil subsets and their gene signature associate with vascular inflammation and coronary atherosclerosis in lupus. JCI Insight 2018;3(8) [pii:99276].

23. Dey AK, Joshi AA, Chaturvedi A, et al. Association between skin and aortic vascular inflammation in patients with psoriasis: a case-cohort study using positron emission tomography/computed tomography. JAMA Cardiol 2017;2(9):1013–8.

24. Geraldino-Pardilla L, Zartoshti A, Ozbek AB, et al. Arterial inflammation detected with (18) F-Fluorodeoxyglucose-Positron emission tomography in rheumatoid arthritis. Arthritis Rheumatol 2018;70(1):30–9.

25. Yarasheski KE, Laciny E, Overton ET, et al. 18FDG PET-CT imaging detects arterial inflammation and early atherosclerosis in HIV-infected adults with cardiovascular disease risk factors. J Inflamm (Lond) 2012;9(1):26.

26. Mehta NN, Yu Y, Saboury B, et al. Systemic and vascular inflammation in patients with moderate to severe psoriasis as measured by [18F]-fluorodeoxyglucose positron emission tomography-computed tomography (FDG-PET/CT): a pilot study. Arch Dermatol 2011;147(9):1031–9.

27. Naik HB, Natarajan B, Stansky E, et al. Severity of psoriasis associates with aortic vascular inflammation detected by FDG PET/CT and neutrophil activation in a prospective observational study. Arterioscler Thromb Vasc Biol 2015;35(12):2667–76.

28. Noh SM, Choi WJ, Kang BT, et al. Complementarity between F-18-FDG PET/CT and ultrasonography or angiography in carotid plaque characterization. J Clin Neurol 2013;9(3):176–85.

29. Kelly PJ, Camps-Renom P, Giannotti N, et al. Carotid plaque inflammation imaged by (18)F-fluorodeoxyglucose positron emission tomography and risk of early recurrent stroke. Stroke 2019;50(7):1766–73.

30. Joshi AA, Lerman JB, Dey AK, et al. Association between aortic vascular inflammation and coronary artery plaque characteristics in psoriasis. JAMA Cardiol 2018;3(10):949–56.

31. Singh P, Emami H, Subramanian S, et al. Coronary plaque morphology and the anti-inflammatory impact of atorvastatin: a multicenter 18F- fluorodeoxyglucose positron emission tomographic/

computed tomographic study. Circ Cardiovasc Imaging 2016;9(12) [pii:e004195].

32. Lee YB, Choi KM. Diet-modulated lipoprotein metabolism and vascular inflammation evaluated by (18)F-fluorodeoxyglucose positron emission tomography. Nutrients 2018;10(10):1382.

33. Tawakol A, Fayad ZA, Mogg R, et al. Intensification of statin therapy results in a rapid reduction in atherosclerotic inflammation: results of a multicenter fluorodeoxyglucose-positron emission tomography/computed tomography feasibility study. J Am Coll Cardiol 2013;62(10):909–17.

34. Lee JL, Sinnathurai P, Buchbinder R, et al. Biologics and cardiovascular events in inflammatory arthritis: a prospective national cohort study. Arthritis Res Ther 2018;20(1):171.

35. Mehta NN, Shin DB, Joshi AA, et al. Effect of 2 psoriasis treatments on vascular inflammation and novel inflammatory cardiovascular biomarkers: a randomized placebo-controlled trial. Circ Cardiovasc Imaging 2018;11(6):e007394.

36. Gelfand JM, Shin DB, Alavi A, Torigian DA, Werner T, Papadopoulos M, et al. A Phase IV, Randomized, Double-Blind, Placebo-Controlled Crossover Study of the Effects of Ustekinumab on Vascular Inflammation in Psoriasis (the VIP-U Trial). Journal of Investigative Dermatology 2020;140(1):85-93.e2.

37. Steinhart CR, Emons MF. Risks of cardiovascular disease in patients receiving antiretroviral therapy for HIV infection: implications for treatment. AIDS Read 2004;14(2):86–90, 93-5.

38. Botkin CD, Osman MM. Prevalence, challenges, and solutions for (18)F-FDG PET studies of obese patients: a technologist's perspective. J Nucl Med Technol 2007;35(2):80–3.

39. Bucerius J, Mani V, Moncrieff C, et al. Optimizing 18F-FDG PET/CT imaging of vessel wall inflammation: the impact of 18F-FDG circulation time, injected dose, uptake parameters, and fasting blood glucose levels. Eur J Nucl Med Mol Imaging 2014;41(2):369–83.

40. Surti S. Update on time-of-flight PET imaging. J Nucl Med 2015;56(1):98–105.

41. Williams G, Kolodny GM. Suppression of myocardial 18F-FDG uptake by preparing patients with a high-fat, low-carbohydrate diet. AJR Am J Roentgenol 2008;190(2):W151–6.

Infection and Inflammation Imaging
Beyond FDG

Malte Kircher, MD, Constantin Lapa, MD*

KEYWORDS

- Inflammation • Infection • PET • Molecular imaging • Somatostatin receptors • CXCR4 • TSPO
- NaF

KEY POINTS

- ^{18}F-FDG PET/CT is the standard of reference in nuclear imaging of infection and inflammation, but lacks specificity.
- Receptor-directed alternatives, such as tracers targeting somatostatin and chemokine receptors on proinflammatory cells have shown promising results in first clinical studies, especially in the setting of myocardial inflammation.
- Many further PET and SPECT probes directed at other specific inflammatory cell receptors, cell adhesion molecules, and proinflammatory cytokines and enzymes are currently being evaluated.

INTRODUCTION

Although inflammation is a crucial and beneficial process in the acute physiologic defense against pathogens, excessive, uncontrolled, or chronic inflammatory reactions can lead to numerous pathologic changes. These include rheumatic and autoimmune diseases, such as rheumatoid arthritis (RA) or vasculitis, as well as several cardiovascular and neurologic disorders.

Traditionally, 3-phase bone scintigraphy, ^{67}Ga-citrate scintigraphy, or white blood cell scintigraphy have been the mainstay of nuclear medicine imaging of inflammation and infection. Nowadays, PET imaging with the glucose analog 2-deoxy-2-[^{18}F] fluoro-D-glucose (^{18}F-FDG, FDG), which takes advantage of the increased glucose metabolism in proinflammatory target cells,[1] is the standard of reference for noninvasive visualization and monitoring of inflammatory processes. However, its nonspecificity and dependence on physiologic variables, such as glucose levels or renal function can limit its suitability in numerous clinical scenarios.

To overcome these shortcomings multiple other tracers have been developed. In this review we discuss nuclear imaging of inflammation using molecular probes beyond FDG and focusing on their cellular targets. Special emphasis is put on diagnostic tracers that have already been successfully applied clinically (**Table 1**).

TARGETING RECEPTORS ON THE CELL SURFACE
Somatostatin Receptor

Somatostatin receptors (SSTR), especially subtype $SSTR_{2A}$, are important diagnostic and therapeutic targets in oncology, with routine use in the management of neuroendocrine tumors and meningiomas. The G protein-coupled receptor can be targeted using synthetic somatostatin analogs, such as 1,4,7,10-tetraazacyclododecane-1,4,7,10-tetraacetic acid (DOTA)-D-Phe-Tyr3-octreotide (DOTA-TOC), DOTA-1-Nal(3)-octreotide (DOTA-NOC), or DOTA-D-Phe-Tyr3-octreotate (DOTA-TATE), which differ mainly in their affinity to the various receptor subtypes ($SSTR_{1-5}$). A particularly rich $SSTR_2$ expression is found on macrophages with numerous studies demonstrating promising results using SSTR-directed PET for detection of various

Department of Nuclear Medicine, University Hospital Augsburg, Stenglinstr. 2, Würzburg 86156, Germany
* Corresponding author.
E-mail address: Constantin.Lapa@uk-augsburg.de

PET Clin 15 (2020) 215–229
https://doi.org/10.1016/j.cpet.2019.11.004

Table 1
PET tracers for inflammation imaging

Target	Tracer	Features
Specific targeting of receptors/transporters/proteins		
Somatostatin receptor (SSTR)	^{68}Ga-DOTA-TOC ^{68}Ga-DOTA-NOC ^{68}Ga-DOTA-TATE	Overexpressed mainly on proinflammatory M1 macrophages. Useful particularly in imaging of cardiac inflammation due to specificity and lack of tracer uptake in healthy myocardium (FDG PET requires the use of dedicated patient preparation strategies to suppress the physiologic myocardial FDG uptake)
C-X-C motif chemokine receptor 4 (CXCR4)	^{68}Ga-Pentixafor	Expressed on a variety of proinflammatory immune cells, with a pronounced overexpression on macrophages and T cells
C-C motif chemokine receptor 2 (CCR2)	^{64}Cu-DOTA ECL1i ^{68}Ga-DOTA ECL1i	Mostly expressed on highly inflammatory monocytes, natural killer cells and T cells
$\alpha_v\beta_3$ integrin receptor	^{18}F-Galacto-RGD ^{68}Ga-PRGD2 ^{18}F-Fluciclatide	Mediates cell adhesion and plays an important role in angiogenesis, making it an interesting target in many different oncologic or inflammatory conditions, such as rheumatoid arthritis
Folate receptor (FR)	^{18}F-Fluoro-PEG-folate	Remarkably high expression on the cell surface of activated macrophages with highly restricted FR expression in normal tissues
Mannose receptor	^{18}F-Fluoro-D-mannose ^{68}Ga-NOTA-HAS ^{68}Ga-NOTA-anti-MMR nanobody	Mainly expressed by macrophages, immature dendritic cells, and liver sinusoidal endothelial cells
Translocator protein-18 kDa (TSPO)	^{11}C-PK11195 and 2nd and 3rd generation TSPO tracers, such as ^{18}F-GE180	Protein situated in the outer mitochondrial membrane; upregulated in activated macrophages, particularly in the brain (microglia). Promising target for neuroinflammation imaging.
Bacterial thymidine kinase	^{124}I-FIAU	Bacteria express a thymidine kinase (TK) that differs from the major human TK in its substrate specificity
Bacterial maltodextrin transporter	^{18}F-Maltohexaose	Bacteria-specific and not found in mammalian cells

(continued on next page)

Table 1
(continued)

Target	Tracer	Features
Unspecific visualization of inflammation		
Proliferation	^{11}C-Methionine	Marker of amino acid transport and protein synthesis, accumulates in inflammatory cells, including macrophages, T cells, and B cells
Proliferation	^{18}F-Fluorothymidine (FLT)	Generally considered a marker of tumor proliferation; able to visualize inflammation with different tracer distribution compared with FDG
Bone metabolism	^{18}F-Sodium flouride (NaF)	Used to assess bone metabolism and osteogenic activity; since NaF also localizes to developing microcalcifications, it can be used as a marker of calcification activity

inflammatory conditions, such as sarcoidosis, myocarditis, or atherosclerosis.

In a study with 20 patients with sarcoidosis, Nobashi and colleagues[2] demonstrated the superiority of ^{68}Ga-DOTA-TOC PET/computed tomography (CT) over ^{67}Ga-scintigraphy for identification of lymph node, uvea, and muscle lesions. Subsequent pilot studies used SSTR-directed PET to detect cardiac sarcoidosis (CS), with results corresponding closely to those of cardiac MR imaging,[3] and outperforming those of ^{18}F-FDG PET.[4] SSTR PET was likewise used to visualize myocardial inflammation in patients with pericarditis, myocarditis, and subacute myocardial infarction (AMI), again with excellent concordance to cardiac MR imaging.[5] Key advantages of SSTR-directed imaging of cardiac inflammation include specific targeting of proinflammatory M1 macrophages,[6] and lack of tracer uptake in healthy myocardium, a significant advantage over ^{18}F-FDG PET, which requires the use of dedicated patient preparation strategies to suppress the physiologic myocardial ^{18}F-FDG uptake.[7–9]

SSTR-directed PET imaging is furthermore capable of localizing inflammation in atherosclerosis. Although initial pilot studies established the general feasibility of this imaging approach in the larger arteries,[10,11] the prospective observational VISION trial, which included 42 patients with acute coronary syndrome and/or transient ischemic attack/stroke, revealed superior imaging characteristics of ^{68}Ga-DOTATATE versus ^{18}F-FDG PET in vessels as small as the coronary arteries[6] (**Fig. 1**). A substudy revealed that SSTR-directed

PET can identify residual postinfarction myocardial inflammation both in recently infarcted myocardium (<3 months) as well as in old ischemic injuries,[12] and also found a strong correlation between bone marrow uptake and myocardial inflammation, which might indicate a potential for noninvasive evaluation of systemic inflammatory networks.[12] Finally, Schatka and colleagues[13] outlined the potential of SSTR-directed peptide receptor radionuclide therapy to alter inflammatory activity in atherosclerotic plaques, a potentially new theranostic approach to modulate plaque biology.

C-X-C Motif Chemokine Receptor 4

C-X-C motif chemokine receptor 4 (CXCR4) is expressed on a variety of proinflammatory immune cells, with a pronounced overexpression on macrophages and T cells. CXCR4-directed PET tracers, such as ^{68}Ga-Pentixafor provide the opportunity to visualize human CXCR4 expression in vivo, and insights from first pilot studies suggest that this approach can contribute to uncovering the highly sophisticated role of chemokines and their receptors in inflammatory processes.

Myocardial inflammation imaging after acute myocardial infarction

Pilot studies that investigated CXCR4-directed PET imaging in the highly inflammatory environment of AMI demonstrated high tracer uptake in the infarcted myocardium[14] (**Fig. 2**), which coincided with the presence of proinflammatory cells in the ischemic area.[15] A further investigation

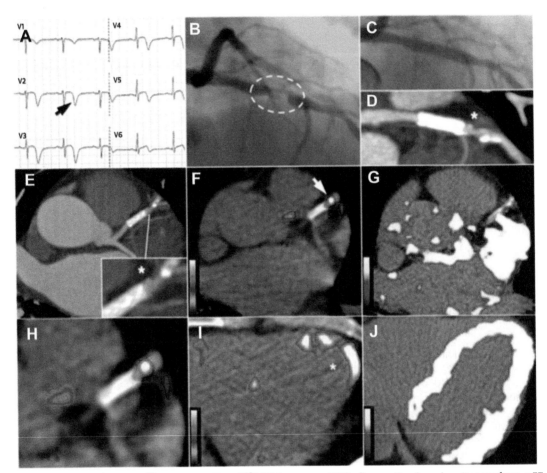

Fig. 1. Comparison between ⁶⁸Ga-DOTATATE and ¹⁸F-FDG coronary PET inflammation imaging. Images from a 57-year-old man with acute coronary syndrome who presented with deep anterolateral T-wave inversion (*arrow*) on electrocardiogram (*A*) and serum troponin-I concentration increased at 4650 ng/L (NR: <17 ng/L). Culprit left anterior descending artery stenosis (dashed oval) was identified by X-ray angiography (*B*). After percutaneous coronary stenting (*C*), residual coronary plaque (*inset) with high-risk morphology (low attenuation and spotty calcification) is evident on CT angiography (*D, E*). ⁶⁸Ga-DOTATATE PET (*F, H, I*) clearly detected intense tracer accumulation in this atherosclerotic plaque/distal portion of the stented culprit lesion (*arrow*) and recently infarcted myocardium (*asterisk*). In contrast, in ¹⁸F-FDG PET (*G, J*), myocardial spillover completely obscures the coronary arteries. CT, computed tomography; ¹⁸F-FDG, fluorine-18-labeled fluorodeoxyglucose; ⁶⁸Ga-DOTATATE, gallium-68-labeled DOTATATE. (*From* Tarkin JM, Joshi FR, Evans NR, et al. Detection of Atherosclerotic Inflammation by (68)Ga-DOTATATE PET Compared to [(18)F]FDG PET Imaging. Journal of the American College of Cardiology. 2017;69(14):1774-1791; with permission.)

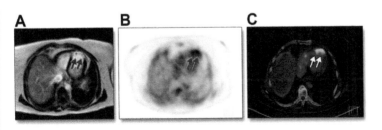

Fig. 2. Increased ⁶⁸Ga-Pentixafor uptake in acute myocardial infarction affecting the left anterior descending artery. Axial slices of both (*A*) contrast-enhanced multishot inversion recovery turbo field echo cardiac MR imaging and (*B*) CXCR4-PET, as well as (*C*) fused PET/computed tomography. Images reveal increased ⁶⁸Ga-Pentixafor uptake in the apex that consistently matches myocardial damage in CMR (*arrows*). (*From* Lapa C, Reiter T, Werner RA, et al. [(68)Ga]Pentixafor-PET/CT for Imaging of Chemokine Receptor 4 Expression After Myocardial Infarction. *JACC Cardiovascular imaging.* 2015;8(12):1466-1468; with permission.)

found a correlation between CXCR4 expression in the bone marrow and the severity of the systemic inflammatory response,[16] and showed that those patients with AMI who had initially high myocardial tracer uptake presented with less scar tissue in the infarcted area and a better functional outcome at follow-up.[16] However, the latter findings are in contradiction with results of a recent preclinical study that reported on beneficial effects of CXCR4 blockade by attenuated inflammatory gene expression via regulatory T cells.[17] More research to broaden our understanding of the spatial and temporal orchestration of CXCR4 expression in the different cell types involved in AMI is highly warranted.

C-X-C motif chemokine receptor 4-directed inflammation imaging in atherosclerosis

At present, a study of 72 patients with lymphoma showed that ^{68}Ga-Pentixafor PET/MRI is able to visualize inflammation within human carotid plaques, with histologic evidence for colocalization of CXCR4 and CD68 in inflamed atheromas and preatheromas.[18] These findings confirmed previous results of CXCR4 overexpression in macrophage-rich plaque regions in a rabbit model of atherosclerosis.[19] In addition, 2 independent studies demonstrated an association between cardiovascular risk factors and CXCR4 expression within atherosclerotic plaques on a per-patient basis, as visualized by ^{68}Ga-Pentixafor PET/CT.[20,21] Derlin and colleagues[22] investigated CXCR4 expression in the coronary arteries of 37 patients with AMI after stent-based reperfusion and found highest ^{68}Ga-Pentixafor uptake in the culprit lesions, which the authors ascribed to vessel wall inflammation and/or stent-induced injury. In another study in patients undergoing CXCR4-directed endoradiotherapy with [177]Lu-/^{90}Y-Pentixather for hematologic malignancy, Li and colleagues[23] were able to show an additional anti-inflammatory therapeutic effect on atherosclerotic plaques.

Whereas most of the PET signal is believed to originate from macrophages, the variety of different cell types expressing the chemokine receptor on their surface (T cells, B cells, and/or progenitor cells) adds complexity to the underlying biology and its clinical implications,[24] and the CXCR4 axis seems to exert both atheroprotective as well as atherogenic, proinflammatory effects.[25,26] This could explain results of a human carotid plaque study that showed CXCR4 overexpression in both stable and unstable atherosclerotic plaques, with the highest receptor expression found on macrophages and macrophage-derived foam cells.[27] Future studies to investigate CXCR4 biology in

atherosclerosis and its clinical implications are highly warranted.

C-X-C motif chemokine receptor 4-directed imaging in infections

Noninvasive targeting of CXCR4 with PET/CT has also been used to image infectious diseases. In a pilot study of 29 patients with suspected chronic osteomyelitis, Bouter and colleagues[28] exploited the increased CXCR4 expression of T cells to successfully visualize inflammatory activity. In a separate study, the same group demonstrated superior diagnostic accuracy of ^{68}Ga-Pentixafor PET/CT for detection of chronic bone infections compared with the granulocyte-directed ^{99m}Tc-besilesomab and ^{99m}Tc-labeled white blood cells.[29] In addition, in an investigation of 13 patients with complicated urinary tract infections after kidney transplantation, infectious foci could successfully be detected by imaging leukocyte infiltration using ^{68}Ga-Pentixafor PET and MRI.[30]

C-C Motif Chemokine Receptor 2

C-C chemokine receptor type 2 (CCR 2; CD 192) is mostly expressed on monocytes, natural killer cells, and T lymphocytes,[31,32] and plays a crucial role in the homeostatic release of monocytes and macrophages from the bone marrow.[33] Interaction of CCR2 with its ligand CCL2 is essential to induce normal inflammatory monocyte migration (from the bone marrow) into peripheral tissues,[34] which is important in the defense against microbial infections. An imbalance in favor of highly inflammatory CCR2[+] macrophages and monocytes can, however, lead to serious pathologic changes and inflammatory conditions, such as atherosclerosis and RA.[35,36] Furthermore, it has been shown that, after AMI, CCR2[+] monocytes infiltrate the heart and differentiate into highly inflammatory CCR2[+] macrophages that ultimately contribute to postinfarction heart failure.[37]

With the development of the allosteric CCR2 ligand "extracellular loop 1 inverso" (ECL1i), noninvasive molecular imaging of CCR2 expression in vivo has become feasible,[38] as illustrated by the results of a pilot study in mice models of cardiac injury that showed accumulation of the new tracer in areas rich in CCR2[+] cells.[39] The authors also provided autoradiographic confirmation of specific tracer binding to human macrophages in heart failure specimens.[39] Another proof-of-concept could be provided in a mouse model of lung injury and in human tissues from subjects with chronic obstructive pulmonary disease.[40] PET using ^{64}Cu-labeled DOTA-ECL1i was able to noninvasively visualize CCR2[+] cells in both mouse lungs (after LPS-induced injury) as well as in human lung disease tissue.[40]

Other Specific Targets

Alpha-v beta-3 receptor

The transmembrane receptor alpha-v beta-3 integrin ($\alpha_v\beta_3$) mediates cell adhesion and plays an important role in angiogenesis, making it an interesting target in many different oncologic or inflammatory conditions.[41,42] Radiopharmaceuticals containing an arginine-glycine-aspartic acid (RGD) sequence, such as ^{18}F-galacto-RGD, ^{68}Ga-PRGD2, and ^{18}F-fluciclatide bind the $\alpha_v\beta_3$ receptor with high affinity and enable noninvasive visualization of $\alpha_v\beta_3$ expression in vivo.[43]

In atherosclerosis, both macrophages and activated endothelial cells have been described to express high levels of the $\alpha_v\beta_3$ receptor.[44,45] Interestingly, the $\alpha_v\beta_3$ integrin may be directly involved in the degradation of the protective fibrous cap of atherosclerotic lesions, because it has been identified as a binding moiety that localizes matrix metalloproteinase 2 to the surface of invasive cells.[46,47] Therefore, $\alpha_v\beta_3$ expression might serve as a potential combined marker of both inflammation and angiogenesis in atherosclerotic lesions and thus as a noninvasive in vivo surrogate parameter of plaque vulnerability.[48] In a study in 10 patients with high-grade carotid artery stenosis, ^{18}F-galacto-RGD uptake significantly correlated with intraplaque $\alpha_v\beta_3$ expression and with results of autoradiography, and could be specifically blocked in in vitro competition experiments. Based on these results, the authors concluded that $\alpha_v\beta_3$-integrin-directed PET visualized several important features of plaque stability that might potentially be advantageous over ^{18}F-FDG.[49] Another study of 21 patients with AMI using the RGD-containing tracer ^{18}F-fluciclatide showed increased tracer uptake in the infarcted area, which the authors attributed to sites of cardiac repair, due to an association between tracer uptake and functional recovery at follow-up.[50] This confirmed results of previous studies with other $\alpha_v\beta_3$-directed PET tracers in a rat model of AMI,[51] and in patients with AMI/stroke.[52]

Apart from cardiovascular imaging, $\alpha_v\beta_3$-directed PET has been used to image conditions associated with angiogenesis, highlighted by a prospectively designed head-to-head comparison between ^{68}Ga-PRGD2 and ^{18}F-FDG PET/CT in 20 patients with untreated RA.[53] The authors demonstrated the superiority of ^{68}Ga-PRGD2 over ^{18}F-FDG for detection and evaluation of severity of active RA lesions and provided histologic confirmation of increased $\alpha_v\beta_3$ expression on neo-endothelial cells of the affected synovia.[53]

Mitochondrial translocator protein

The 18-kDa mitochondrial translocator protein (TSPO) is a 5-transmembrane domain protein situated in the outer mitochondrial membrane and is widely distributed in most peripheral organs, including kidneys, nasal epithelium, adrenal glands, lungs, and heart.[54] In contrast, due to minimal expression in resting microglial cells, it has been found to be a promising target for neuroinflammation imaging.[55] Because TSPO is also upregulated in activated macrophages, its use might be extended to the visualization of non-neurologic, peripheral inflammatory processes as well as the characterization of systemic inflammatory responses, for example, the heart-brain axis after myocardial infarction.

In a series of trials of patients with RA, TSPO-directed PET was able to detect subclinical synovitis via imaging of activated macrophages, even when MRI was inconspicuous.[56–59] In studies in the setting of atherosclerosis and vascular inflammation in patients with systemic inflammatory disorders, the selective TSPO ligand ^{11}C-PK11195 was able to visualize activated macrophages in the vessel wall and improve cerebrovascular risk stratification.[60–62] Of note, TSPO PET detected inflammatory activity even in asymptomatic patients and might therefore prove a useful tool for very early disease detection. However, some limitations of TSPO PET tracers for the detection of peripheral inflammatory conditions, such as its multicellular receptor expression profile, the presence of radiolabeled metabolites and an interindividual variability of tracer binding affinity due to TSPO polymorphisms have to be taken into account.[63] Beyond these drawbacks, strengths of TSPO-directed PET imaging are the ability to visualize both central and peripheral inflammatory networks and the interplay between activated microglia and macrophages, as highlighted in a recent study by Thackeray and colleagues.[64] In a mouse model of AMI the authors revealed that, in addition to the inflammatory response in the infarcted myocardium, there was an interaction between systemic inflammatory networks and neuronal inflammation via activated microglia (**Fig. 3**). These results could be corroborated in 3 patients after AMI, thus highlighting the systemic interaction between heart and brain after cardiac ischemia. A pilot study in patients with controlled HIV infection also hinted at the suitability of TSPO PET to depict concomitant neuroinflammation.[65]

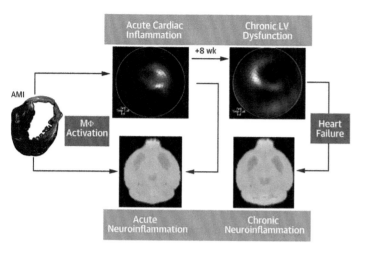

Fig. 3. Serial imaging demonstrating concurrent increase of TSPO in the heart and brain after acute MI and in chronic heart failure. Distribution of the mitochondrial translocator protein (TSPO) ligand ^{18}F-GE180 denotes inflammation in the heart and brain after acute myocardial infarction. Perfusion-corrected ^{18}F-GE180 polar map shows increased TSPO expression in the anterolateral infarct territory at 1 week post-MI, associated with increased TSPO and neuroinflammation. After 8 weeks and the development of heart failure, TSPO is increased in the remote myocardium with recurrent neuroinflammation proportional to the decline in cardiac function. AMI, acute myocardial infarction; MΦ, macrophage. (*From* Thackeray JT, Hupe HC, Wang Y, et al. Myocardial Inflammation Predicts Remodeling and Neuroinflammation After Myocardial Infarction. Journal of the American College of Cardiology. 2018;71(3):263-275; with permission.)

Folate receptor

Folate receptor beta (FR-β) is a glycosyl-phosphatidylinositol-anchored protein that binds the vitamin folic acid with high affinity and internalizes it via endocytosis.[66] Except for an overexpression on proximal tubule cells in the kidneys, FR prevalence is limited in normal tissues. However, a remarkably high FR expression on the surface of activated macrophages has been described,[67] and FRs have been targeted to study inflammatory conditions, such as RA. An example is a study by Gent and colleagues[68] in a rat model of RA that demonstrated superiority of ^{18}F-fluoro-PEG-folate over the mitochondrial translocator protein PET tracer PK11195 for detection of RA. In another study, FR-targeted PET was able to identify affected joints in patients with RA and provided histologic proof from synovial tissue samples.[69] Numerous other preclinical studies are currently evaluating the potential of targeting the FR-β for diagnosis and treatment of inflammatory diseases (mainly RA).[70,71]

Mannose receptor

The mannose receptor (CD206) is mainly expressed by macrophages, immature dendritic cells, and liver sinusoidal endothelial cells,[72] and several preclinical studies have already evaluated the possibility of targeting it for inflammation imaging. For example, ^{18}F-fluoro-D-mannose PET/CT was used in a rabbit model to identify inflammation within atherosclerotic plaques,[73] whereas ^{68}Ga-NOTA-mannosylated human serum albumin (MSA) PET was successfully utilized in different animal models for detection of inflammation in atherosclerotic

plaques and myocarditis, respectively.[74,75] Recently, a study in apoE-knock out mice demonstrated feasibility of atherosclerotic plaque imaging by visualization of (M2a) macrophages using a ^{68}Ga-labeled anti-MR-nanobody.[76]

Thymidine kinase

Bacteria express a thymidine kinase (TK) that differs from the major human TK in its substrate specificity. This was exploited by Diaz and colleagues[77] who used [124]I-labeled 1-(2′-deoxy-2′-fluoro-b-D-arabinofuranosyl)-5-iodouracil (FIAU), a substrate of the bacteria TK, to detect musculoskeletal infections in a pilot study with 8 patients. But despite these promising results, the whole-body distribution with significant uptake in liver, kidneys, muscles, and to a lesser extent in several other organs, potentially due to the presence of a mitochondrial enzyme resembling the bacterial TK, raised concerns about the general applicability of the tracer. These concerns were reaffirmed in a study on [124]I-FIAU PET for detection of prosthetic joint infections that revealed low specificity and sensitivity of the tracer.[78]

Maltodextrin transporter

The bacteria-specific maltodextrin transporter is not found in mammalian cells and can be targeted with ^{18}F-labeled maltohexaose (^{18}F-MH). Ning and colleagues[79] showed in rats that ^{18}F-MH PET can identify early stage infections consisting of as few as 10^5 colony-forming units of *E. coli*. In a recent investigation using a model of *Staphylococcus aureus*-mediated infections associated with implanted cardiac devices, ^{18}F-MH but not ^{18}F-FDG PET was able to distinguish infection from noninfectious inflammation.[80] Thus, this new imaging probe holds great potential for the translation of bacterial imaging in humans.

Other targeted tracers

Numerous other imaging probes have been investigated that cannot be extensively covered in this review, including receptor-directed tracers that target immune cells, such as T lymphocytes (CD3 and CD4) and B lymphocytes (CD20), or granulocytes (BW250/183),[81] as well as tracers for specific noninvasive imaging of bacterial infections. For a comprehensive overview over the current literature and most promising candidates for infection-specific PET imaging of bacteria, please refer to the review by Auletta and colleagues.[82]

TARGETING CELL PROLIFERATION AND CELL METABOLISM

As an alternative to receptor-directed imaging, tracers targeting increased inflammatory cell metabolism have been evaluated. Although these tracers are obviously not inflammation specific, they may offer advantages over ^{18}F-FDG in certain scenarios, for example, for the assessment of inflammatory heart processes, such as myocarditis or sarcoidosis, due to the absence of physiologic uptake in the healthy myocardium.

Methionine

The radiolabeled amino acid L-[methyl-^{11}C]methionine (^{11}C-methionine) as a marker of amino acid transport and protein synthesis is predominantly used in oncology, particularly for the imaging of brain tumors and multiple myeloma.[83–87] However, methionine uptake is also increased in monocytes and macrophages that migrate to sites of inflammatory activity.[88,89] In vitro binding experiments using isolated inflammatory cells confirmed that ^{14}C-methionine accumulates in inflammatory cells, including macrophages, T cells, and B cells,[90] suggesting the applicability of ^{11}C-methionine PET for detection of inflammatory lesions, especially in the setting after acute ischemia. In a pilot study of 9 patients with AMI, Morooka and colleagues[91] demonstrated increased myocardial ^{11}C-methionine uptake in the infarct area, with reduced or no uptake in ^{18}F-FDG PET and ^{201}Tl perfusion SPECT, respectively. Thackeray and colleagues[92] confirmed these results by tracing ^{11}C-methionine accumulation in the infarcted area back to inflammatory M1 macrophages using a mouse model and 1 human patient. Increased uptake of ^{11}C-methionine was also found in inflammatory lesions of a rat model with induced autoimmune inflammatory myocarditis.[93]

Fluorothymidine

3′-Deoxy-3′-^{18}F-fluorothymidine (FLT) has been mostly evaluated in the oncologic setting as a marker of tumor proliferation. FLT is transported into the cell by nucleoside transporters, phosphorylated by thymidine kinase 1 (which is particularly active between the late G1 and early G2 phase of the cell cycle), and subsequently trapped within the cell.[94] Thus, FLT also holds promise as a tracer to image inflammation by depicting cell proliferation.

In a mouse model of experimental RA, FLT PET/CT revealed enhanced tracer uptake in inflamed ankles as early as 1 day after arthritis induction. Imaging findings correlated strongly with immunohistochemical Ki67 staining and was therefore considered a promising tool for the in vivo assessment of arthritic joint inflammation.[95] Clinical experience with FLT is currently growing for sarcoidosis. Norikane and colleagues[96] studied 20 patients with sarcoidosis, who underwent both FLT and FDG PET/CT. FLT was able to identify CS and extracardiac lesions, but tracer uptake was lower as compared with FDG. Recently, a pilot study reported on an equally excellent performance of FLT PET in the detection of CS as compared with FDG. Interestingly, the distribution pattern of the 2 tracers in the myocardium differed, suggesting a distinct pathophysiological source of the respective signal.[97] Further research including of the value of FLT PET as a biomarker for CS is warranted.

Sodium Fluoride

PET imaging with sodium ^{18}F-fluoride (NaF) has been extensively used to assess bone metabolism and osteogenic activity.[98] Because NaF also localizes to developing microcalcifications, it can be used as a marker of calcification activity and has been investigated in a range of cardiovascular disorders including aortic stenosis or atherosclerosis, and other inflammatory conditions, such as RA. In an experimental mouse model of RA, NaF PET identified sites of enhanced pathologic bone metabolism in diseased joints. In addition, the PET signal significantly correlated with the degree of bone destruction.[99] A study comparing NaF and FDG PET in 12 patients with RA found a similar distribution pattern of both tracers, with NaF PET being able to successfully identify RA-affected joints.[100]

Many studies have been performed for the evaluation of NaF PET for the characterization of vascular wall microcalcifications and could confirm the feasibility of this approach for large (aorta), carotid, and even coronary arteries.[101–104]

We refer to recent reviews for more detailed information.[105,106] Of note, the NaF PET signal did not colocalize with morphologic calcification (as detected by CT) or vessel wall inflammation (as detected by FDG PET) in a significant number of cases, suggesting that all modalities target distinct biological processes and stages in atherosclerosis. Beyond mere identification of sites of active calcification, NaF PET might serve as a noninvasive biomarker of increased cardiovascular risk. Among neurologically asymptomatic oncology patients undergoing NaF PET/CT, tracer accumulation in the common carotid arteries was correlated with cardiovascular risk factors and carotid calcified plaque burden.[101] In patients after recent transient ischemic attack or minor ischemic stroke, NaF PET was equally useful to highlight culprit and high-risk carotid plaques.[107] The predictive value of NaF PET could be confirmed for coronary atherosclerotic plaques (with NaF, but not FDG PET) and thoracic aorta calcification (with patients exhibiting high NaF uptake being prone to a 3.7 times higher cardiovascular disease risk based on the Framingham risk score)[108] as well as for symptomatic peripheral arterial disease (with NaF uptake demonstrating excellent discrimination in predicting 1-year restenosis after lower limb percutaneous transluminal angioplasty).[109] In contrast to these encouraging results, the suitability of NaF PET to detect active CS needs to be determined.[110]

OTHER TRACERS

Numerous PET tracers have been developed and are being evaluated for the purpose of infection and inflammation imaging, including tracers targeting most antibiotics, adhesion molecules, such as members of the integrin and selectin family, the immunoglobulin superfamily, or cytokines and enzymes, for example, matrix metalloproteinase or tumor necrosis factor alpha.[81]

Vascular adhesion protein-1 is a glycoprotein on endothelial cells and is involved in the transfer of leukocytes from blood to tissues on inflammation.[111] Several promising radiolabeled antibodies and peptides have been assessed.[111–115]

Selectins are single-chain transmembrane glycoproteins and are classified into 3 subtypes (L-, E–, and P-selectins) depending on the cell type on which they originate.[116] P-selectin is located in the α-granules of platelets and is expressed by activated endothelia.[117] Thus, it can be used as a target for imaging atherosclerosis, and radiolabeled probes for imaging P-selectin including Fucoidan have been assessed in preclinical models.[118–120]

The P2X7 receptor, a member of the purinergic family of receptors, is an adenosine triphosphate-gated ion channel expressed predominantly on macrophages and monocytes in the periphery and on microglia and astrocytes in the central nervous system. Because of its widespread involvement in inflammatory diseases as a key regulatory element of the inflammasome complex, with initiation and sustenance of the inflammatory cascade, it has attracted some attention and various SPECT and PET tracers have been evaluated.[121–126] In a recent inflammation versus tumor model in mice, the ^{18}F-labeled PsX7 tracer ^{18}F-PTTP (5-1-pyrimidin-2-yl-4,5,6,7-tetrahydro-1H-[1,2,3]triazolo[4,5-c]pyridin) showed promise to differentiate inflammation from malignancy.[127]

Another promising target is fibroblast activation protein (FAP), a 170-kDa transmembrane glycoprotein that has dipeptidyl peptidase and endopeptidase activity and shows high upregulation in epithelial carcinoma and sites of tissue remodeling, including fibrosis and arthritis.[128] Several radiolabeled antibodies have been used to target and image FAP expression in malignant and inflamed tissues, particularly in RA.[129–132] Recently, PET tracers based on small-molecule enzyme inhibitors have become clinically available.[133,134]

Various studies have looked at nanoparticles that are internalized by macrophages through phagocytosis.[135] Keliher and colleagues[136] were able to visualize cardiovascular inflammation in mice and rabbits using an ^{18}F-labeled, modified polyglucose nanoparticle called Macroflor with high avidity for macrophages.

SUMMARY

^{18}F-FDG PET/CT is by far the most established tracer in nuclear medicine infection and inflammation imaging and has proven its value in various clinical settings including fever of unknown origin,[137] endocarditis,[138] or sarcoidosis.[139] However, the glucose analog FDG is taken up by almost any metabolically active tissue, limiting its specificity for detecting inflammatory cells. In fact, in the setting of atherosclerosis, microautoradiography studies of aortic sections of ApoE$^{-/-}$ mice have shown that ^{14}C-FDG uptake into atherosclerotic plaques correlates poorly with fat content and selective macrophage staining with anti-CD68.[140] In addition, persistent vascular FDG uptake in patients with clinically controlled arteritis could not always reliably identify the subjects at risk to relapse,[141] thus raising concerns about the utility of FDG PET in the

follow-up of vasculitis and rendering its use to monitor disease activity controversial.[142]

Moreover, physiologic tracer uptake can severely impair the diagnostic performance in some scenarios (e.g. CS) requiring dedicated patient preparation.[143]

To overcome these limitations, many—potentially more specific—alternatives for noninvasive infection and inflammation imaging have been explored. At present, the clinically best established compounds target SSTRs on the cell surface of M1 macrophages, with a growing body of evidence suggesting the superiority of the SSTR-directed approach, particularly in coronary arteries.[6]

Many other monocyte-/macrophage-targeting tracers, such as mannose receptor, CCR2, or P2X7, have demonstrated encouraging preclinical results but need to be further assessed in clinical trials.

In atherosclerosis, detection of active calcification by means of NaF PET/CT is gaining growing attention.

Another clinically established option includes imaging of CXCR4 that holds potential for the detection of systemic inflammatory networks and could be especially used to monitor receptor-directed therapies, for example, after AMI. However, given the high abundance of different CXCR4-expressing cell types, further research investigating the different sources of the PET signal in different conditions is still needed until firm conclusions on the value of chemokine receptor-directed PET imaging can be drawn. The same holds true for most other promising compounds that have shown encouraging results in specific scenarios but are to be fully validated until their routine use instead of or complimentary to ^{18}F-FDG can be recommended.

CONFLICTS OF INTERESTS

The authors declare no conflicts of interest.

REFERENCES

1. Meller J, Sahlmann CO, Scheel AK. ^{18}F-FDG PET and PET/CT in fever of unknown origin. J Nucl Med 2007;48(1):35–45.
2. Nobashi T, Nakamoto Y, Kubo T, et al. The utility of PET/CT with (68)Ga-DOTATOC in sarcoidosis: comparison with (67)Ga-scintigraphy. Ann Nucl Med 2016;30(8):544–52.
3. Lapa C, Reiter T, Kircher M, et al. Somatostatin receptor based PET/CT in patients with the suspicion of cardiac sarcoidosis: an initial comparison to cardiac MRI. Oncotarget 2016;7(47):77807–14.
4. Gormsen LC, Haraldsen A, Kramer S, et al. A dual tracer (68)Ga-DOTANOC PET/CT and (18)F-FDG PET/CT pilot study for detection of cardiac sarcoidosis. EJNMMI Res 2016;6(1):52.
5. Lapa C, Reiter T, Li X, et al. Imaging of myocardial inflammation with somatostatin receptor based PET/CT—a comparison to cardiac MRI. Int J Cardiol 2015;194:44–9.
6. Tarkin JM, Joshi FR, Evans NR, et al. Detection of atherosclerotic inflammation by (68)Ga-DOTATATE PET compared to [(18)F]FDG PET imaging. J Am Coll Cardiol 2017;69(14):1774–91.
7. Harisankar CN, Mittal BR, Agrawal KL, et al. Utility of high fat and low carbohydrate diet in suppressing myocardial FDG uptake. J Nucl Cardiol 2011;18(5):926–36.
8. Williams G, Kolodny GM. Suppression of myocardial 18F-FDG uptake by preparing patients with a high-fat, low-carbohydrate diet. AJR Am J Roentgenol 2008;190(2):W151–6.
9. Ishimaru S, Tsujino I, Takei T, et al. Focal uptake on ^{18}F-fluoro-2-deoxyglucose positron emission tomography images indicates cardiac involvement of sarcoidosis. Eur Heart J 2005;26(15):1538–43.
10. Li X, Bauer W, Kreissl MC, et al. Specific somatostatin receptor II expression in arterial plaque: (68)Ga-DOTATATE autoradiographic, immunohistochemical and flow cytometric studies in apoE-deficient mice. Atherosclerosis 2013;230(1):33–9.
11. Li X, Samnick S, Lapa C, et al. ^{68}Ga-DOTATATE PET/CT for the detection of inflammation of large arteries: correlation with ^{18}F-FDG, calcium burden and risk factors. EJNMMI Res 2012;2(1):52.
12. Tarkin JM, Calcagno C, Dweck MR, et al. 68)Ga-DOTATATE PET identifies residual myocardial inflammation and bone marrow activation after myocardial infarction. J Am Coll Cardiol 2019;73(19):2489–91.
13. Schatka I, Wollenweber T, Haense C, et al. Peptide receptor-targeted radionuclide therapy alters inflammation in atherosclerotic plaques. J Am Coll Cardiol 2013;62(24):2344–5.
14. Lapa C, Reiter T, Werner RA, et al. [(68)Ga]Pentixafor-PET/CT for imaging of chemokine receptor 4 expression after myocardial infarction. JACC Cardiovasc Imaging 2015;8(12):1466–8.
15. Thackeray JT, Derlin T, Haghikia A, et al. Molecular imaging of the chemokine receptor CXCR4 after acute myocardial infarction. JACC Cardiovasc Imaging 2015;8(12):1417–26.
16. Reiter T, Kircher M, Schirbel A, et al. Imaging of C-X-C motif chemokine receptor CXCR4 expression after myocardial infarction with [(68)Ga]Pentixafor-PET/CT in correlation with cardiac MRI. JACC Cardiovasc Imaging 2018;11(10):1541–3.
17. Wang Y, Dembowsky K, Chevalier E, et al. C-X-C motif chemokine receptor 4 blockade promotes

tissue repair after myocardial infarction by enhancing regulatory T cell mobilization and immune-regulatory function. Circulation 2019; 139(15):1798–812.

18. Li X, Yu W, Wollenweber T, et al. [(68)Ga]Pentixafor PET/MR imaging of chemokine receptor 4 expression in the human carotid artery. Eur J Nucl Med Mol Imaging 2019;46(8):1616–25.

19. Hyafil F, Pelisek J, Laitinen I, et al. Imaging the cytokine receptor CXCR4 in atherosclerotic plaques with the radiotracer (68)Ga-pentixafor for PET. J Nucl Med 2017;58(3):499–506.

20. Li X, Heber D, Leike T, et al. [68Ga]Pentixafor-PET/MRI for the detection of Chemokine receptor 4 expression in atherosclerotic plaques. Eur J Nucl Med Mol Imaging 2018;45(4):558–66.

21. Weiberg D, Thackeray JT, Daum G, et al. Clinical molecular imaging of chemokine receptor CXCR4 expression in atherosclerotic plaque using (68) Ga-pentixafor PET: correlation with cardiovascular risk factors and calcified plaque burden. J Nucl Med 2018;59(2):266–72.

22. Derlin T, Sedding DG, Dutzmann J, et al. Imaging of chemokine receptor CXCR4 expression in culprit and nonculprit coronary atherosclerotic plaque using motion-corrected [(68)Ga]pentixafor PET/CT. Eur J Nucl Med Mol Imaging 2018; 45(11):1934–44.

23. Li X, Kemmer L, Zhang X, et al. Anti-inflammatory effects on atherosclerotic lesions induced by CXCR4-directed endoradiotherapy. J Am Coll Cardiol 2018;72(1):122–3.

24. Pawig L, Klasen C, Weber C, et al. Diversity and inter-connections in the CXCR4 chemokine receptor/ligand family: molecular perspectives. Front Immunol 2015;6:429.

25. van der Vorst EP, Doring Y, Weber C. MIF and CXCL12 in cardiovascular diseases: functional differences and similarities. Front Immunol 2015;6:373.

26. Doring Y, Pawig L, Weber C, et al. The CXCL12/CXCR4 chemokine ligand/receptor axis in cardiovascular disease. Front Physiol 2014;5:212.

27. Merckelbach S, van der Vorst EPC, Kallmayer M, et al. Expression and cellular localization of CXCR4 and CXCL12 in human carotid atherosclerotic plaques. Thromb Haemost 2018;118(1):195–206.

28. Bouter Y, Meller B, Sahlmann CO, et al. Immunohistochemical detection of chemokine receptor 4 expression in chronic osteomyelitis confirms specific uptake in 68Ga-Pentixafor-PET/CT. Nuklearmedizin 2018;57(5):198–203.

29. Bouter C, Meller B, Sahlmann CO, et al. 68)Ga-Pentixafor PET/CT imaging of chemokine receptor CXCR4 in chronic infection of the bone: first insights. J Nucl Med 2018;59(2):320–6.

30. Derlin T, Gueler F, Brasen JH, et al. Integrating MRI and chemokine receptor CXCR4-targeted PET for detection of leukocyte infiltration in complicated urinary tract infections after kidney transplantation. J Nucl Med 2017;58(11):1831–7.

31. Charo IF, Ransohoff RM. The many roles of chemokines and chemokine receptors in inflammation. N Engl J Med 2006;354(6):610–21.

32. Tomankova T, Kriegova E, Liu M. Chemokine receptors and their therapeutic opportunities in diseased lung: far beyond leukocyte trafficking. Am J Physiol Lung Cell Mol Physiol 2015;308(7):L603–18.

33. Shi C, Pamer EG. Monocyte recruitment during infection and inflammation. Nat Rev Immunol 2011;11(11):762–74.

34. Griffith JW, Sokol CL, Luster AD. Chemokines and chemokine receptors: positioning cells for host defense and immunity. Annu Rev Immunol 2014;32:659–702.

35. Raghu H, Lepus CM, Wang Q, et al. CCL2/CCR2, but not CCL5/CCR5, mediates monocyte recruitment, inflammation and cartilage destruction in osteoarthritis. Ann Rheum Dis 2017;76(5):914–22.

36. Verweij SL, Duivenvoorden R, Stiekema LCA, et al. CCR2 expression on circulating monocytes is associated with arterial wall inflammation assessed by 18F-FDG PET/CT in patients at risk for cardiovascular disease. Cardiovasc Res 2018;114(3):468–75.

37. Bajpai G, Schneider C, Wong N, et al. The human heart contains distinct macrophage subsets with divergent origins and functions. Nat Med 2018;24(8):1234–45.

38. Auvynet C, Baudesson de Chanville C, Hermand P, et al. ECL1i, d(LGTFLKC), a novel, small peptide that specifically inhibits CCL2-dependent migration. FASEB J 2016;30(6):2370–81.

39. Heo GS, Kopecky B, Sultan D, et al. Molecular imaging visualizes recruitment of inflammatory monocytes and macrophages to the injured heart. Circ Res 2019;124(6):881–90.

40. Liu Y, Gunsten SP, Sultan DH, et al. PET-based imaging of chemokine receptor 2 in experimental and disease-related lung inflammation. Radiology 2017;283(3):758–68.

41. Brooks PC, Clark RA, Cheresh DA. Requirement of vascular integrin alpha v beta 3 for angiogenesis. Science 1994;264(5158):569–71.

42. Brooks PC, Montgomery AM, Rosenfeld M, et al. Integrin alpha v beta 3 antagonists promote tumor regression by inducing apoptosis of angiogenic blood vessels. Cell 1994;79(7):1157–64.

43. Dijkgraaf I, Beer AJ, Wester HJ. Application of RGD-containing peptides as imaging probes for alphavbeta3 expression. Front Biosci (Landmark Ed) 2009;14:887–99.

44. Hoshiga M, Alpers CE, Smith LL, et al. Alpha-v beta-3 integrin expression in normal and atherosclerotic artery. Circ Res 1995;77(6):1129–35.

45. Antonov AS, Kolodgie FD, Munn DH, et al. Regulation of macrophage foam cell formation by alphaVbeta3 integrin: potential role in human atherosclerosis. Am J Pathol 2004;165(1):247–58.

46. van Hinsbergh VW, Engelse MA, Quax PH. Pericellular proteases in angiogenesis and vasculogenesis. Arterioscler Thromb Vasc Biol 2006;26(4):716–28.

47. Brooks PC, Stromblad S, Sanders LC, et al. Localization of matrix metalloproteinase MMP-2 to the surface of invasive cells by interaction with integrin alpha v beta 3. Cell 1996;85(5):683–93.

48. Razavian M, Marfatia R, Mongue-Din H, et al. Integrin-targeted imaging of inflammation in vascular remodeling. Arterioscler Thromb Vasc Biol 2011;31(12):2820–6.

49. Beer AJ, Pelisek J, Heider P, et al. PET/CT imaging of integrin alphavbeta3 expression in human carotid atherosclerosis. JACC Cardiovasc Imaging 2014;7(2):178–87.

50. Jenkins WS, Vesey AT, Stirrat C, et al. Cardiac alphaVbeta3 integrin expression following acute myocardial infarction in humans. Heart 2017;103(8):607–15.

51. Higuchi T, Bengel FM, Seidl S, et al. Assessment of alphavbeta3 integrin expression after myocardial infarction by positron emission tomography. Cardiovasc Res 2008;78(2):395–403.

52. Sun Y, Zeng Y, Zhu Y, et al. Application of (68)Ga-PRGD2 PET/CT for alphavbeta3-integrin imaging of myocardial infarction and stroke. Theranostics 2014;4(8):778–86.

53. Zhu Z, Yin Y, Zheng K, et al. Evaluation of synovial angiogenesis in patients with rheumatoid arthritis using (6)(8)Ga-PRGD2 PET/CT: a prospective proof-of-concept cohort study. Ann Rheum Dis 2014;73(6):1269–72.

54. Banati RB. Visualising microglial activation in vivo. Glia 2002;40(2):206–17.

55. Dupont AC, Largeau B, Santiago Ribeiro MJ, et al. Translocator protein-18 kDa (TSPO) positron emission tomography (PET) imaging and its clinical impact in neurodegenerative diseases. Int J Mol Sci 2017;18(4) [pii:E785].

56. van der Laken CJ, Elzinga EH, Kropholler MA, et al. Noninvasive imaging of macrophages in rheumatoid synovitis using 11C-(R)-PK11195 and positron emission tomography. Arthritis Rheum 2008;58(11):3350–5.

57. Gent YY, Voskuyl AE, Kloet RW, et al. Macrophage positron emission tomography imaging as a biomarker for preclinical rheumatoid arthritis: findings of a prospective pilot study. Arthritis Rheum 2012;64(1):62–6.

58. Gent YY, Ter Wee MM, Voskuyl AE, et al. Subclinical synovitis detected by macrophage PET, but not MRI, is related to short-term flare of clinical disease activity in early RA patients: an exploratory study. Arthritis Res Ther 2015;17:266.

59. Gent YY, Ahmadi N, Voskuyl AE, et al. Detection of subclinical synovitis with macrophage targeting and positron emission tomography in patients with rheumatoid arthritis without clinical arthritis. J Rheumatol 2014;41(11):2145–52.

60. Pugliese F, Gaemperli O, Kinderlerer AR, et al. Imaging of vascular inflammation with [^{11}C]-PK11195 and positron emission tomography/computed tomography angiography. J Am Coll Cardiol 2010;56(8):653–61.

61. Lamare F, Hinz R, Gaemperli O, et al. Detection and quantification of large-vessel inflammation with ^{11}C-(R)-PK11195 PET/CT. J Nucl Med 2011;52(1):33–9.

62. Gaemperli O, Shalhoub J, Owen DR, et al. Imaging intraplaque inflammation in carotid atherosclerosis with 11C-PK11195 positron emission tomography/computed tomography. Eur Heart J 2012;33(15):1902–10.

63. Owen DR, Yeo AJ, Gunn RN, et al. An 18-kDa translocator protein (TSPO) polymorphism explains differences in binding affinity of the PET radioligand PBR28. J Cereb Blood flow Metab 2012;32(1):1–5.

64. Thackeray JT, Hupe HC, Wang Y, et al. Myocardial inflammation predicts remodeling and neuroinflammation after myocardial infarction. J Am Coll Cardiol 2018;71(3):263–75.

65. Vera JH, Guo Q, Cole JH, et al. Neuroinflammation in treated HIV-positive individuals: a TSPO PET study. Neurology 2016;86(15):1425–32.

66. Muller C. Folate based radiopharmaceuticals for imaging and therapy of cancer and inflammation. Curr Pharm Des 2012;18(8):1058–83.

67. Salazar MD, Ratnam M. The folate receptor: what does it promise in tissue-targeted therapeutics? Cancer Metastasis Rev 2007;26(1):141–52.

68. Gent YY, Weijers K, Molthoff CF, et al. Evaluation of the novel folate receptor ligand [^{18}F]fluoro-PEG-folate for macrophage targeting in a rat model of arthritis. Arthritis Res Ther 2013;15(2):R37.

69. Xia W, Hilgenbrink AR, Matteson EL, et al. A functional folate receptor is induced during macrophage activation and can be used to target drugs to activated macrophages. Blood 2009;113(2):438–46.

70. Chandrupatla D, Molthoff CFM, Lammertsma AA, et al. The folate receptor beta as a macrophage-mediated imaging and therapeutic target in rheumatoid arthritis. Drug Deliv Transl Res 2019;9(1):366–78.

71. Hu Y, Wang B, Shen J, et al. Depletion of activated macrophages with a folate receptor-beta-specific

antibody improves symptoms in mouse models of rheumatoid arthritis. Arthritis Res Ther 2019;21(1): 143.

72. Martinez-Pomares L. The mannose receptor. J Leukoc Biol 2012;92(6):1177–86.

73. Tahara N, Mukherjee J, de Haas HJ, et al. 2-Deoxy-2-[18F]fluoro-D-mannose positron emission tomography imaging in atherosclerosis. Nat Med 2014; 20(2):215–9.

74. Lee SP, Im HJ, Kang S, et al. Noninvasive imaging of myocardial inflammation in myocarditis using (68)Ga-tagged mannosylated human serum albumin positron emission tomography. Theranostics 2017;7(2):413–24.

75. Kim EJ, Kim S, Seo HS, et al. Novel PET imaging of atherosclerosis with 68Ga-labeled NOTA-neomannosylated human serum albumin. J Nucl Med 2016;57(11):1792–7.

76. Varasteh Z, Mohanta S, Li Y, et al. Targeting mannose receptor expression on macrophages in atherosclerotic plaques of apolipoprotein E-knockout mice using (68)Ga-NOTA-anti-MMR nanobody: non-invasive imaging of atherosclerotic plaques. EJNMMI Res 2019;9(1):5.

77. Diaz LA Jr, Foss CA, Thornton K, et al. Imaging of musculoskeletal bacterial infections by [124I]FIAU-PET/CT. PLoS One 2007;2(10):e1007.

78. Zhang XM, Zhang HH, McLeroth P, et al. [(124)I]FIAU: human dosimetry and infection imaging in patients with suspected prosthetic joint infection. Nucl Med Biol 2016;43(5):273–9.

79. Ning X, Seo W, Lee S, et al. PET imaging of bacterial infections with fluorine-18-labeled maltohexaose. Angew Chem Int Ed Engl 2014;53(51): 14096–101.

80. Takemiya K, Ning X, Seo W, et al. Novel PET and near infrared imaging probes for the specific detection of bacterial infections associated with cardiac devices. JACC Cardiovasc Imaging 2019;12(5):875–86.

81. Lee HJ, Ehlerding EB, Cai W. Antibody-based tracers for PET/SPECT imaging of chronic inflammatory diseases. Chembiochem 2019;20(4): 422–36.

82. Auletta S, Varani M, Horvat R, et al. PET radiopharmaceuticals for specific bacteria imaging: a systematic review. J Clin Med 2019;8(2) [pii:E197].

83. Herholz K, Holzer T, Bauer B, et al. 11C-Methionine PET for differential diagnosis of low-grade gliomas. Neurology 1998;50(5):1316–22.

84. Kracht LW, Miletic H, Busch S, et al. Delineation of brain tumor extent with [11C]L-methionine positron emission tomography: local comparison with stereotactic histopathology. Clin Cancer Res 2004; 10(21):7163–70.

85. Lapa C, Garcia-Velloso MJ, Luckerath K, et al. 11)C-Methionine-PET in multiple myeloma: a combined study from two different institutions. Theranostics 2017;7(11):2956–64.

86. Luckerath K, Lapa C, Albert C, et al. 11C-Methionine-PET: a novel and sensitive tool for monitoring of early response to treatment in multiple myeloma. Oncotarget 2015;6(10):8418–29.

87. Luckerath K, Lapa C, Spahmann A, et al. Targeting paraprotein biosynthesis for non-invasive characterization of myeloma biology. PLoS One 2013; 8(12):e84840.

88. Swirski FK, Nahrendorf M. Leukocyte behavior in atherosclerosis, myocardial infarction, and heart failure. Science 2013;339(6116):161–6.

89. Nahrendorf M. Myeloid cell contributions to cardiovascular health and disease. Nat Med 2018;24(6): 711–20.

90. Oka S, Okudaira H, Ono M, et al. Differences in transport mechanisms of trans-1-amino-3-[18F]fluorocyclobutanecarboxylic acid in inflammation, prostate cancer, and glioma cells: comparison with L-[methyl-11C]methionine and 2-deoxy-2-[18F]fluoro-D-glucose. Mol Imaging Biol 2014;16(3): 322–9.

91. Morooka M, Kubota K, Kadowaki H, et al. 11C-Methionine PET of acute myocardial infarction. J Nucl Med 2009;50(8):1283–7.

92. Thackeray JT, Bankstahl JP, Wang Y, et al. Targeting amino acid metabolism for molecular imaging of inflammation early after myocardial infarction. Theranostics 2016;6(11):1768–79.

93. Maya Y, Werner RA, Schutz C, et al. 11C-Methionine PET of myocardial inflammation in a rat model of experimental autoimmune myocarditis. J Nucl Med 2016;57(12):1985–90.

94. Herrmann K, Buck AK. Proliferation imaging with (1)(8)F-fluorothymidine PET/computed tomography: physiologic uptake, variants, and pitfalls. PET Clin 2014;9(3):331–8.

95. Fuchs K, Kohlhofer U, Quintanilla-Martinez L, et al. In vivo imaging of cell proliferation enables the detection of the extent of experimental rheumatoid arthritis by 3'-deoxy-3'-18F-fluorothymidine and small-animal PET. J Nucl Med 2013;54(1):151–8.

96. Norikane T, Yamamoto Y, Maeda Y, et al. Comparative evaluation of (18)F-FLT and (18)F-FDG for detecting cardiac and extra-cardiac thoracic involvement in patients with newly diagnosed sarcoidosis. EJNMMI Res 2017;7(1):69.

97. Martineau P, Pelletier-Galarneau M, Juneau D, et al. Imaging cardiac sarcoidosis with FLT-PET with comparison to FDG-PET: a prospective pilot study. J Nucl Med 2019;60(Suppl 1):670.

98. Blau M, Nagler W, Bender MA. Fluorine-18: a new isotope for bone scanning. J Nucl Med 1962;3: 332–4.

99. Irmler IM, Gebhardt P, Hoffmann B, et al. 18F-Fluoride positron emission tomography/computed tomography

for noninvasive in vivo quantification of pathophysiological bone metabolism in experimental murine arthritis. Arthritis Res Ther 2014;16(4):R155.

100. Watanabe T, Takase-Minegishi K, Ihata A, et al. 18)F-FDG and (18)F-NaF PET/CT demonstrate coupling of inflammation and accelerated bone turnover in rheumatoid arthritis. Mod Rheumatol 2016;26(2):180–7.

101. Derlin T, Wisotzki C, Richter U, et al. In vivo imaging of mineral deposition in carotid plaque using ¹⁸F-sodium fluoride PET/CT: correlation with atherogenic risk factors. J Nucl Med 2011;52(3):362–8.

102. Derlin T, Richter U, Bannas P, et al. Feasibility of ¹⁸F-sodium fluoride PET/CT for imaging of atherosclerotic plaque. J Nucl Med 2010;51(6): 862–5.

103. Li Y, Berenji GR, Shaba WF, et al. Association of vascular fluoride uptake with vascular calcification and coronary artery disease. Nucl Med Commun 2012;33(1):14–20.

104. Dweck MR, Chow MW, Joshi NV, et al. Coronary arterial ¹⁸F-sodium fluoride uptake: a novel marker of plaque biology. J Am Coll Cardiol 2012;59(17): 1539–48.

105. Silva Mendes BI, Oliveira-Santos M, Vidigal Ferreira MJ. Sodium fluoride in cardiovascular disorders: a systematic review. J Nucl Cardiol 2019. https://doi.org/10.1007/s12350-019-01832-7.

106. McKenney-Drake ML, Moghbel MC, Paydary K, et al. (18)F-NaF and (18)F-FDG as molecular probes in the evaluation of atherosclerosis. Eur J Nucl Med Mol Imaging 2018;45(12):2190–200.

107. Vesey AT, Jenkins WS, Irkle A, et al. (18)F-Fluoride and (18)F-fluorodeoxyglucose positron emission tomography after transient ischemic attack or minor ischemic stroke: case-control study. Circ Cardiovasc Imaging 2017;10(3) [pii:e004976].

108. Blomberg BA, de Jong PA, Thomassen A, et al. Thoracic aorta calcification but not inflammation is associated with increased cardiovascular disease risk: results of the CAMONA study. Eur J Nucl Med Mol Imaging 2017;44(2):249–58.

109. Chowdhury MM, Tarkin JM, Albaghdadi MS, et al. Vascular positron emission tomography and restenosis in symptomatic peripheral arterial disease: a prospective clinical study. JACC Cardiovasc Imaging 2019. https://doi.org/10.1016/j.jcmg.2019.03.031.

110. Weinberg RL, Morgenstern R, DeLuca A, et al. F-18 sodium fluoride PET/CT does not effectively image myocardial inflammation due to suspected cardiac sarcoidosis. J Nucl Cardiol 2017;24(6):2015–8.

111. Moisio O, Siitonen R, Liljenback H, et al. Exploring alternative radiolabeling strategies for sialic acid-binding immunoglobulin-like lectin 9 peptide: [(68)Ga]Ga- and [(18)F]AlF-NOTA-Siglec-9. Molecules 2018;23(2) [pii:E305].

112. Lankinen P, Makinen TJ, Poyhonen TA, et al. (68)Ga-DOTAVAP-P1 PET imaging capable of demonstrating the phase of inflammation in healing bones and the progress of infection in osteomyelitic bones. Eur J Nucl Med Mol Imaging 2008;35(2): 352–64.

113. Autio A, Vainio PJ, Suilamo S, et al. Preclinical evaluation of a radioiodinated fully human antibody for in vivo imaging of vascular adhesion protein-1-positive vasculature in inflammation. J Nucl Med 2013;54(8):1315–9.

114. Autio A, Henttinen T, Sipila HJ, et al. Mini-PEG spaceing of VAP-1-targeting 68Ga-DOTAVAP-P1 peptide improves PET imaging of inflammation. EJNMMI Res 2011;1(1):10.

115. Aalto K, Autio A, Kiss EA, et al. Siglec-9 is a novel leukocyte ligand for vascular adhesion protein-1 and can be used in PET imaging of inflammation and cancer. Blood 2011;118(13):3725–33.

116. McMurray RW. Adhesion molecules in autoimmune disease. Semin Arthritis Rheum 1996;25(4): 215–33.

117. Ley K. The role of selectins in inflammation and disease. Trends Mol Med 2003;9(6):263–8.

118. Li X, Bauer W, Israel I, et al. Targeting P-selectin by gallium-68-labeled fucoidan positron emission tomography for noninvasive characterization of vulnerable plaques: correlation with in vivo 17.6T MRI. Arterioscler Thromb Vasc Biol 2014;34(8): 1661–7.

119. Nakamura I, Hasegawa K, Wada Y, et al. Detection of early stage atherosclerotic plaques using PET and CT fusion imaging targeting P-selectin in low density lipoprotein receptor-deficient mice. Biochem Biophys Res Commun 2013;433(1):47–51.

120. Xu Y, Li J, Fang W, et al. A potential thrombus diagnosis reagent based on P-selectin monoclonal antibody SZ-51 light chain. Thromb Res 2008;123(2): 306–15.

121. Kolb HC, Barret O, Bhattacharya A, et al. Preclinical evaluation and nonhuman primate receptor occupancy study of (18)F-JNJ-64413739, a PET radioligand for P2X7 receptors. J Nucl Med 2019; 60(8):1154–9.

122. Territo PR, Meyer JA, Peters JS, et al. Characterization of (11)C-GSK1482160 for targeting the P2X7 receptor as a biomarker for neuroinflammation. J Nucl Med 2017;58(3):458–65.

123. Ory D, Celen S, Gijsbers R, et al. Preclinical evaluation of a P2X7 receptor-selective radiotracer: PET studies in a rat model with local overexpression of the human P2X7 receptor and in nonhuman primates. J Nucl Med 2016;57(9):1436–41.

124. Fantoni ER, Dal Ben D, Falzoni S, et al. Design, synthesis and evaluation in an LPS rodent model of neuroinflammation of a novel (18)F-labelled PET tracer targeting P2X7. EJNMMI Res 2017;7(1):31.

125. Jin H, Han J, Resing D, et al. Synthesis and in vitro characterization of a P2X7 radioligand [(123)I]TZ6019 and its response to neuroinflammation in a mouse model of Alzheimer disease. Eur J Pharmacol 2018;820:8–17.

126. Janssen B, Vugts DJ, Wilkinson SM, et al. Identification of the allosteric P2X7 receptor antagonist [(11)C]SMW139 as a PET tracer of microglial activation. Sci Rep 2018;8(1):6580.

127. Fu Z, Lin Q, Hu B, et al. P2X7 PET radioligand (18)F-PTTP for differentiation of lung tumor from inflammation. J Nucl Med 2019;60(7):930–6.

128. Hamson EJ, Keane FM, Tholen S, et al. Understanding fibroblast activation protein (FAP): substrates, activities, expression and targeting for cancer therapy. Proteomics Clin Appl 2014;8(5–6):454–63.

129. Welt S, Divgi CR, Scott AM, et al. Antibody targeting in metastatic colon cancer: a phase I study of monoclonal antibody F19 against a cell-surface protein of reactive tumor stromal fibroblasts. J Clin Oncol 1994;12(6):1193–203.

130. Terry SY, Koenders MI, Franssen GM, et al. Monitoring therapy response of experimental arthritis with radiolabeled tracers targeting fibroblasts, macrophages, or integrin alphavbeta3. J Nucl Med 2016;57(3):467–72.

131. Laverman P, van der Geest T, Terry SY, et al. Immuno-PET and immuno-SPECT of rheumatoid arthritis with radiolabeled anti-fibroblast activation protein antibody correlates with severity of arthritis. J Nucl Med 2015;56(5):778–83.

132. van der Geest T, Laverman P, Gerrits D, et al. Liposomal treatment of experimental arthritis can be monitored noninvasively with a radiolabeled anti-fibroblast activation protein antibody. J Nucl Med 2017;58(1):151–5.

133. Loktev A, Lindner T, Mier W, et al. A tumor-imaging method targeting cancer-associated fibroblasts. J Nucl Med 2018;59(9):1423–9.

134. Lindner T, Loktev A, Altmann A, et al. Development of quinoline-based theranostic ligands for the targeting of fibroblast activation protein. J Nucl Med 2018;59(9):1415–22.

135. Majmudar MD, Yoo J, Keliher EJ, et al. Polymeric nanoparticle PET/MR imaging allows macrophage detection in atherosclerotic plaques. Circ Res 2013;112(5):755–61.

136. Keliher EJ, Ye YX, Wojtkiewicz GR, et al. Polyglucose nanoparticles with renal elimination and macrophage avidity facilitate PET imaging in ischaemic heart disease. Nat Commun 2017;8:14064.

137. Kouijzer IJE, Mulders-Manders CM, Bleeker-Rovers CP, et al. Fever of unknown origin: the value of FDG-PET/CT. Semin Nucl Med 2018;48(2):100–7.

138. Mahmood M, Kendi AT, Ajmal S, et al. Meta-analysis of 18F-FDG PET/CT in the diagnosis of infective endocarditis. J Nucl Cardiol 2019;26(3):922–35.

139. Piekarski E, Benali K, Rouzet F. Nuclear imaging in sarcoidosis. Semin Nucl Med 2018;48(3):246–60.

140. Matter CM, Wyss MT, Meier P, et al. 18F-Choline images murine atherosclerotic plaques ex vivo. Arterioscler Thromb Vasc Biol 2006;26(3):584–9.

141. Blockmans D, de Ceuninck L, Vanderschueren S, et al. Repetitive 18F-fluorodeoxyglucose positron emission tomography in giant cell arteritis: a prospective study of 35 patients. Arthritis Rheum 2006;55(1):131–7.

142. Yamashita H, Kubota K, Mimori A. Clinical value of whole-body PET/CT in patients with active rheumatic diseases. Arthritis Res Ther 2014;16(5):423.

143. Ramirez R, Trivieri M, Fayad ZA, et al. Advanced imaging in cardiac sarcoidosis. J Nucl Med 2019;60(7):892–8.

Novel Quantitative PET Imaging Techniques in Tuberculosis

Viplav Deogaonkar, MBBS[a], Bangkim Chandra Khangembam, MD, FANMB[b],
Siavash Mehdizadeh Seraj, MD[a], Abass Alavi, MD[a],
Rakesh Kumar, MD, PhD[c],*, Mboyo-di-tamba Vangu, MD, MMed[d],
Gregory Bisson, MD, MSCE[e]

KEYWORDS

• Quantification • Tuberculosis • Global assessment • FDG • PET/CT

KEY POINTS

- PET/computed tomography (CT) can be readily applied to the assessment of the disease extent and treatment response in tuberculosis (TB) patients.
- The quantitative analysis of PET/CT has succeeded in the assessment of disease burden and treatment response monitoring.
- The accuracy and precision of PET quantification can be improved by adopting new quantitative techniques that are able to reflect the total disease activity.

INTRODUCTION

Globally, an estimated 10 million new patients developed tuberculosis (TB) in 2018, of which around 1.2 million people (among human immunodeficiency virus [HIV] negative) and 251,000 (among HIV positive), respectively, died.[1,2] Caused by the organism *Mycobacterium tuberculosis*, TB is now the leading cause of death from a single infectious agent (ranking above HIV/AIDS).[1] Multidrug-resistant (MDR)-TB occurs because of a selection of mutations in *M tuberculosis*, which leads to resistance to first-line anti-TB agents like isoniazid and rifampicin.[3] MDR-TB incidence has continued to increase, with as many as 558,000 new cases with resistance to rifampicin in 2017. Of these, 82% were found to have MDR-TB, and about 8.5% of the MDR-TB cases were found to be extensively drug resistant (XDR-TB).[1,4] Thus, with TB posing such a threat to the health of the general population, it becomes imperative to diagnose and treat it as early as possible. Many imaging modalities exist for the diagnosis and follow-up of TB, each having its own benefits and drawbacks. PET with ^{18}F-fluorodeoxyglucose (^{18}F-FDG-PET) as an imaging modality has been explored for diagnosis as well as for assessing the treatment response in TB[5]; however, it has its own drawbacks.[6] In order to overcome these drawbacks, the authors discuss the evolving role of hybrid ^{18}F-FDG-PET computed tomography (CT) imaging (FDG-PET/CT) in TB and describe novel quantitative imaging techniques in the diagnosis and assessment of treatment response in TB.

[a] Department of Radiology, Hospital of University of Pennsylvania, Philadelphia, PA 19104, USA;
[b] Department of Nuclear Medicine, All India Institute of Medical Sciences, New Delhi 110029, India;
[c] Diagnostic Nuclear Medicine Division, All India Institute of Medical Sciences, New Delhi 110029, India;
[d] Department of Nuclear Medicine, University of Johannesburg, PO Box 524, Auckland Park 2006, South Africa; [e] Center for Clinical Epidemiology and Biostatistics, University of Pennsylvania, Philadelphia, PA 19104-602, USA
* Corresponding author.
E-mail address: rkphulia@yahoo.com

PET Clin 15 (2020) 231–240
https://doi.org/10.1016/j.cpet.2019.11.010

PET IMAGING AND TRACERS

Similar to the mechanism of conventional glucose uptake, FDG uptake is seen in cells with high metabolic activity.[7] The radiotracer thus accumulates within the inflammatory cells, such as neutrophils and macrophages. The accumulation can be quantified and is measured as a standardized uptake value (SUV).[8] This property of ^{18}F-FDG uptake in cells with high metabolic activity has made it the tracer of choice for use in oncology,[8] and it has also been explored for detection, assessment of disease activity, staging, as well as management of infective-inflammatory diseases, such as TB.[9] ^{18}F-FDG-PET/CT provides a whole-body image, which can be used pretherapeutically to assess the burden of the disease as well as posttherapeutically in assessing the response to treatment.[10] However, 1 significant drawback of using ^{18}F-FDG-PET in infectious diseases like TB is its lack of specificity,[10] which can be improved by combining it with CT imaging.[11,12] Because of increased uptake being shown by lung nodules in cancer as well as TB, it becomes difficult to differentiate between the two.[13] The tracer ^{11}C-choline has helped overcome this drawback, because when combined with ^{18}F-FDG, it helps distinguish TB from malignancy and may also play a pivotal role in therapy management. ^{68}Ga-citrate has been postulated to be better than CT for detecting extrapulmonary lesions. Other than these clinically approved tracers, current research is focused in the preclinical stage on other tracers, such as ^{18}F-sodium fluoride, ^{11}C-pyrazinamide, ^{11}C-isoniazid, and ^{11}C-rifampicin.[13]

ASSESSING DISEASE EXTENT AND DISEASE BURDEN
Pulmonary Tuberculosis

The lungs are the most commonly involved organs in TB,[6] with most patients presenting with pulmonary complaints, such as cough with blood and sputum.[1] Many countries still rely on sputum smear microscopy for the diagnosis of TB; however, because of a sensitivity of only about 50%, most cases can go undetected. It is also not possible to measure drug sensitivity with sputum smear microscopy.[1,10] For these reasons, imaging modalities may be used in conjunction with sputum smear microscopy, with chest radiograph being the most commonly used in diagnosis as well as in follow-up. However, with chest radiograph having shown a diagnostic accuracy of only 49% for pulmonary TB,[10] other imaging techniques such as CT and ^{18}F-FDG-PET/CT are being explored in the diagnosis and management of pulmonary TB.

Li and colleagues[14] conducted a comparative study in 96 patients between PET, CT, and PET/CT imaging to measure their diagnostic accuracy in detecting benign/malignant solitary pulmonary nodules in areas with a high incidence of pulmonary TB. The study concluded that PET/CT imaging had a higher accuracy as compared with PET or CT imaging alone, with 57% of false positives in PET occurring because of TB.[14] ^{18}F-FDG-PET alone therefore cannot be used to differentiate between malignancies and pulmonary TB.[11,15,16] The tracer ^{68}Ga-alfatide has been shown to be superior to ^{18}F-FDG in diagnosing non–small cell lung carcinoma (NSCLC) from pulmonary TB in a study conducted by Kang and colleagues[17] in 34 patients. However, validation of PET/CT imaging with studies that assess a greater number of subjects is needed before it can be used routinely in clinical practice.

Besides having higher sensitivity for diagnosing pulmonary TB, ^{18}F-FDG-PET/CT has been shown to detect latent TB in the subclinical stage.[8] ^{18}F-FDG-PET/CT has shown very high sensitivity as well as specificity in differentiating active pulmonary TB from inactive pulmonary tuberculomas with an SUVmax cutoff of 1.05 at 1-hour intervals.[10] This finding appears important because treatment of latent TB can reduce the number of overt TB cases which can result from reactivation or recent exposure.[18] ^{18}F-FDG-PET/CT imaging has helped in identifying 2 predominant patterns of lung involvement in TB: the predominant lung pattern and the predominant lymphatic pattern. The predominant lung pattern shows pulmonary symptoms with parenchymal involvement, whereas the predominant lymphatic pattern has been shown to be more commonly associated with extrapulmonary TB involvement. The development of these patterns, as shown by Ankrah and colleagues,[10] depends on host immunity at the time of infection with TB. Patients with better immunity show the predominant lung pattern, whereas those who are immunodeficient show the predominant lymphatic pattern.[10,19] Thus, it may help in predicting the type of involvement likely to be seen in patients, which can have significant impact in improving management of patients. **Fig. 1** shows the disease extent in a known case of pulmonary TB.

Lung inflammation as detected by PET/CT is also being considered as a potential marker for predicting the progression of latent to active infection.[10] With TB ranging from latent disease to active disease, it becomes important to identify if the latent disease will progress to active disease because that would significantly alter the management of such patients. Higher ^{18}F-FDG uptake in old TB lesions has been found to correlate with a higher risk

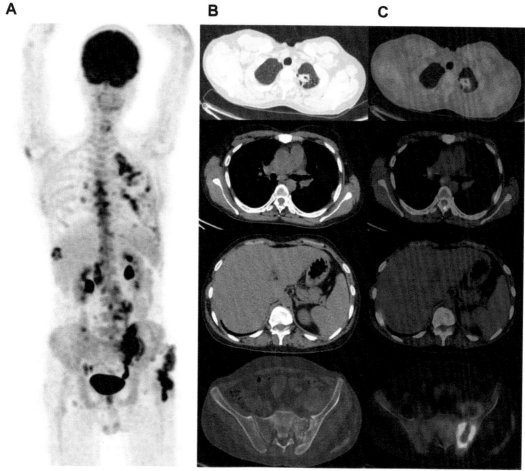

Fig. 1. A 27-year-old man with pulmonary TB for baseline evaluation. 18F-FDG-PET/CT reveals FDG avid cavitary lesion in the apicoposterior segment of left lung upper lobe with multiple fibronodular lesions in the left lung, multiple bilateral parenchymal nodules, bilateral pleural thickening, multiple mediastinal lymph nodes, abdominopelvic lymph nodes, multiple skeletal sites, including left iliac bone, left sacral ala, sacroiliac joint, right knee joint (not shown), along with cold abscesses involving the paraspinal muscles of lumbar region, left iliopsoas muscles, and left gluteal region. (*A*) Maximum intensity projection (MIP) image; (*B*) CT images; (*C*) fused PET/CT images.

for TB reactivation. However, studies are still ongoing, with factors such as total lung ^{18}F-FDG avidity, SUVmax of the most intense latent TB infection granuloma present, size of the largest granuloma, cumulative ^{18}F-FDG avidity on metabolically active mediastinal lymph nodes, and the number of extrapulmonary TB sites being assessed.[10]

Extrapulmonary Tuberculosis

The most frequently involved sites for extrapulmonary TB include lymph nodes, peritoneum, ileocecal junction, liver-spleen, and the genitourinary, musculoskeletal, and central nervous systems.[20] Almost 1 in every 5 patients with TB presents with extrapulmonary TB involvement. As mentioned earlier, immunodeficient patients have

a higher risk of extrapulmonary involvement. Therefore, radiological investigations play an important role in diagnosing extrapulmonary involvement, with MR imaging and CT scans being used more commonly. However, ^{18}F-FDG-PET/CT imaging has seen an upward trend in use because it can show changes at the molecular level,[10,20] as compared with CT and MR imaging scans. The molecular data provided by PET may have important implications in the management of patients.

^{18}F-FDG-PET/CT has been used for assessing generalized lymphadenopathy.[21–23] In tubercular lymphadenopathy, ^{18}F-FDG-PET/CT shows a central hypometabolism with a peripheral uptake, depending on the degree of caseation.[20] Although it has a high sensitivity in detecting lymphadenopathy because of infectious causes like TB, a high number of false positives may be seen because of its inability to differentiate between malignant and benign lymphadenopathy. However, in patients with diagnosed TB or high clinical suspicion of TB, it can help in assessing disease extent, including extrapulmonary lymph node involvement, and also can help as a guide site for biopsy for confirmation of TB.

After lymphadenitis, pleural TB is the most common extrapulmonary site of involvement. Sun and colleagues[24] concluded that ^{18}F-FDG-PET/CT is a more reliable modality in distinguishing malignant from benign pleural effusion. The study showed a specificity of 92.6% in 176 patients, which was much more than either ^{18}F-FDG-PET or CT imaging alone.

Studies[11,25,26] have been conducted regarding the use of ^{18}F-FDG-PET/CT imaging in abdominal sites of TB involvement, such as the stomach, peritoneum, liver, adrenals, and pancreas. Of these, only the use in differentiating between TB peritonitis and peritoneal carcinomatosis showed statistical significance.[27] However, more studies in larger populations need to be conducted for a better understanding of the use of ^{18}F-FDG-PET/CT imaging in abdominal involvement. **Fig. 2**

shows the disease extent in a known case of extrapulmonary TB.

Studies[10,20,28] assessing the utility of ^{18}F-FDG-PET/CT in musculoskeletal involvement have reported that ^{18}F-FDG-PET/CT imaging can be used as a complementary imaging modality to MR imaging, which shows the necessary anatomic structure and involvement in TB. Although individual use of this technique has not been suggested, ^{18}F-FDG-PET/CT has shown increased uptake in tubercular spondylitis, which can help in identifying the multiple sites of involvement as well as in offering support in adequate management.[20,28] The biggest advantage is that ^{18}F-FDG-PET/CT can be used even in the presence of metallic implants, whereas CT imaging gets affected by metal artifacts and MR imaging cannot be used in such patients altogether.[29] However, further studies assessing the utility of ^{18}F-FDG-PET/CT imaging in TB involving the musculoskeletal system need to be undertaken on a larger patient population.

With regard to TB involvement of the central nervous system, Gambhir and colleagues[30] showed that ^{18}F-FDG-PET/CT can help in assessing the disease burden. When compared with MR imaging, radiographs, and ultrasound imaging,

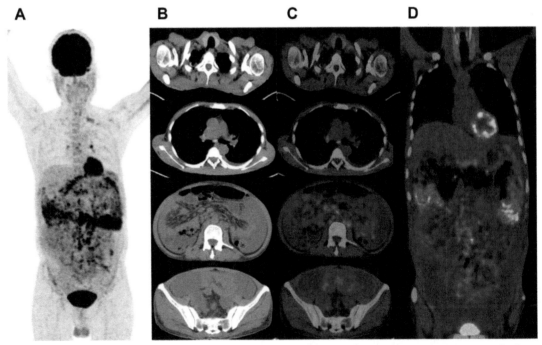

Fig. 2. A 46-year-old man with abdominal TB diagnosed from omental biopsy undergoing FDG-PET/CT for baseline evaluation. FDG-PET/CT reveals active disease involving bilateral supraclavicular, left internal mammary, and multiple abdominal lymph nodes and omentum along with associated small left-sided pleural effusion and gross ascites. (*A*) MIP image; (*B*) CT images; (*C*) fused axial FDG-PET/CT images; (*D*) fused coronal FDG-PET/CT image showing omental involvement and abdominal lymph nodes.

^{18}F-FDG-PET/CT imaging showed a greater sensitivity in detecting extracranial tubercular lesions, which had previously been missed with the other imaging modalities.[30] However, again, studies with a large patient population need to be conducted in order for a better understanding and to derive a definitive role. For intracranial lesions and brain abscesses, ^{18}F-FDG-PET/CT imaging showed a lower sensitivity because of its physiologic uptake by the brain.

When used for TB involvement of the heart, ^{18}F-FDG-PET/CT imaging proved useful for detecting pericarditis in 2 case reports as published by Testempassi and colleagues.[31] They also claimed that in addition to diagnosing the extrapulmonary pericardial involvement in TB, ^{18}F-FDG-PET/CT imaging also helped in directing the treatment.[31]

The conclusions of these studies show the emerging role ^{18}F-FDG-PET/CT imaging in assessing extrapulmonary TB as well as the need to conduct more studies to define a concrete role that can be played by ^{18}F-FDG-PET/CT imaging.

TREATMENT RESPONSE EVALUATION

Even though there is a widespread use of an attenuated live vaccine and the availability of multiple antituberculous drugs,[32] treatment of TB is a big challenge, because it is hard to differentiate patients with drug-sensitive TB from those with drug-resistant TB, which may be MDR-TB or XDR-TB. Patients with MDR-TB are resistant to all first-line drugs, whereas XDR-TB patients are resistant to first-line and some second-line antituberculous drugs. A new entity with resistance to all

antituberculous drugs has also come up recently, labeled as superextensive drug-resistant TB.[13] For these reasons, it has become imperative to come up with techniques that can help identify the drug-resistance status of the patient's disease and then modify the treatment according to the response shown to the medications, rather than the current blanket 6-month regimen for drug-sensitive TB[33,34] or 18- to 24-month regimen for MDR-TB.[34]

^{18}F-FDG-PET imaging has been suggested for this because of its property of showing images at the molecular level. A study conducted by Demura and colleagues[35] compared the uptake of ^{18}F-FDG in pulmonary mycobacteriosis (with 25 out of 47 patients suffering from TB) before and after initiating treatment. The findings suggested that, in comparison to the pretreatment scan, SUVs were lower in patients who were treatment responsive as well as when compared with those who were treatment unresponsive.[35]

Similarly, a study conducted by Martinez and colleagues[36] in 21 patients with TB (pulmonary or extrapulmonary) showed findings pointing toward the use of ^{18}F-FDG-PET/CT imaging as a noninvasive imaging modality for early assessment of the response to antituberculous drugs. More recently, Chen and colleagues[37] assessed the relationship between PET/CT findings and treatment outcomes in MDR-TB patients. Of the 35 subjects enrolled in the study, 24 patients were treatment successes, with PET/CT imaging showing a higher sensitivity in predicting the 6-month treatment response on imaging at 2 months. However, the increase in sensitivity and specificity as compared with that of sputum culture at 2 months was not

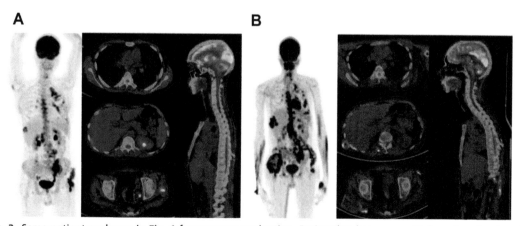

Fig. 3. Same patient as shown in **Fig. 1** for response evaluation. Patient has been on antituberculous treatment (ATT) for 5 months. FDG-PET/CT reveals disease progression in multiple previously seen lesions along with development of multiple new lesions, including new pleural involvement, right chest wall, and right gluteal lesions. (*A*) Baseline scan; (*B*) follow-up scan after 5 months of ATT.

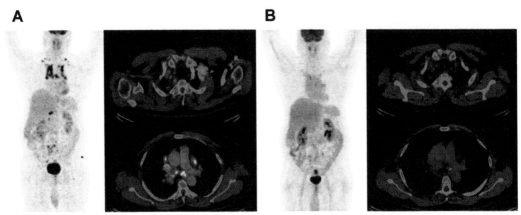

Fig. 4. A 43-year-old man with TB of mediastinal lymph nodes for response evaluation after 3 months of ATT. Baseline FDG-PET/CT (*A*) reveals active disease involving the left supraclavicular, right infraclavicular, and multiple mediastinal lymph nodes. Follow-up FDG-PET/CT (*B*) reveals significant reduction in the size and activity of the involved lymph nodes suggestive of good response to treatment.

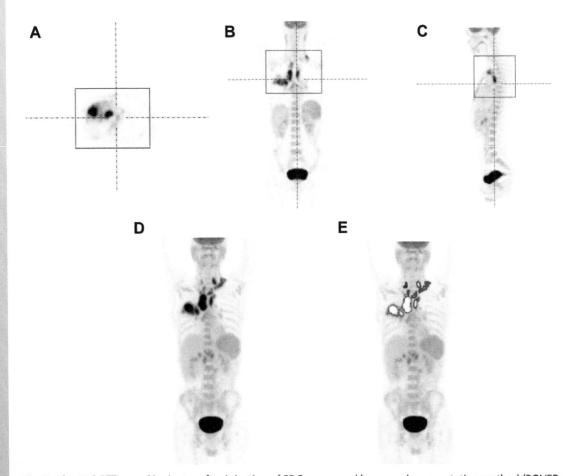

Fig. 5. The FDG-PET scans 60 minutes after injection of FDG as assessed by a novel segmentation method (ROVER; ABX, Radeberg, Germany). A single square-shaped mask was placed on the axial (*A*), coronal (*B*), and sagittal (*C*) planes of the PET image (*D*). The adaptive contrast-oriented thresholding algorithm of ROVER calculated various PET parameters (*E*) The adaptive contrast-oriented thresholding algorithm of ROVER (SUVmean: 10.4; pvcSUV-mean: 16.6; SUVmax: 21.2; volume: 90.8; TLG: 944.1; pvcTLG: 1504.4). (*Courtesy of* M.D. Vangu, MD, University of the Witwatersrand, Johannesburg.)

statistically significant, which could have been due to the low power (32%) of the study. In conclusion, the study claimed that the differences will be more significantly highlighted with a higher sample size for such a study. **Figs. 3** and **4** show response evaluations in 2 patients.

In 2018, a study was conducted by Choi and colleagues[38] on 4 MDR-TB patients, who underwent serial FDG-PET/CT scanning at baseline, and 6 months and 12 months after treatment. The study used average SUV (SUVmean), SUVmax, total metabolic lung volume (sum of metabolic volumes from the hypermetabolic parenchymal lesions), and total lesion glycolysis (TLG; sum of lesion glycolysis from the hypermetabolic parenchymal lesions, see later discussion) as the measured parameters in PET. The study found a significant association between pretreatment volume-based ^{18}F-FDG-PET/CT lung parameters with the final therapeutic response in patients with pulmonary MDR-TB.[38]

However, the biggest drawback of all these studies is the limited sample sizes and heterogeneity. Further studies on a larger patient population are encouraged with ^{18}F-FDG-PET/CT

imaging done before initiating treatment and during different stages of treatment, and then the findings should be compared and analyzed in drug-sensitive as well as in drug-resistant TB patients.

NOVEL QUANTITATIVE IMAGING TECHNIQUES

Quantitative imaging with ^{18}F-FDG-PET/CT has assumed great importance in clinical oncology in the past 2 decades.[39] Conventionally, SUVmax and SUVmean have been used as the characteristics for assessing ^{18}F-FDG uptake in quantitative imaging.[40–42] However, other parameters, such as maximum tumor volume (MTV), TLG, and partial-volume-corrected TLG (pvc-TLG), are also being used in oncology.[41,43–47]

Salavati and colleagues[43] demonstrated that pretherapeutic volumetric quantitative analysis of the whole-body and primary tumor site in NSCLC patients was strongly prognostic of overall survival of such patients. The analyzed PET parameters included SUVmax, SUVmean, MTV, and TLG. The study suggested that if the volumetric quantitative analysis of these characteristics crossed an

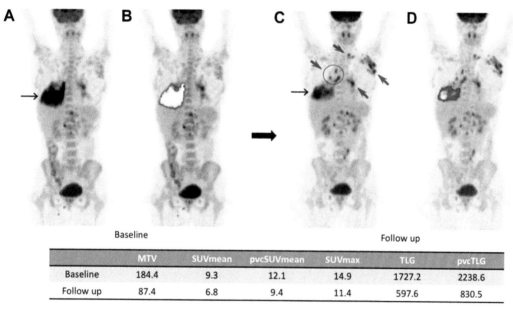

	MTV	SUVmean	pvcSUVmean	SUVmax	TLG	pvcTLG
Baseline	184.4	9.3	12.1	14.9	1727.2	2238.6
Follow up	87.4	6.8	9.4	11.4	597.6	830.5

Fig. 6. Baseline (*A, B*) and follow-up (*C, D*) MIP PET images of an HIV/TB-positive patient. The lung lesion decreased in size and disease activity following 2 months of antiretroviral therapy (*black arrows*). Coincident with response to treatment in the lung lesion, an increased lymph node reaction was observed on FDG-PET scan (*red arrows*). The FDG-avid lung inflammatory site was segmented semiautomatically using an adaptive contrast-oriented thresholding system (ROVER; ABX). The values for metabolic tumor volume (MTV), SUVmean, partial volume-corrected SUVmean (pvcSUVmean), SUVmax, total lesion glycolysis (TLG), and partial volume-corrected total lesion glycolysis (pvcTLG) at the baseline and the follow-up are noted in the table. (*From* Alavi A, Hess S, Werner TJ, et al. An update on the unparalleled impact of FDG-PET imaging on the day-to-day practice of medicine with emphasis on management of infectious/inflammatory disorders. Eur J Nucl Med Mol Imaging. 2019 Sep 4. doi: 10.1007/s00259-019-04490-6. These images are courtesy of Professor Mboyo-Di-Tamba Vangu, University of the Witwatersrand, Johannesburg.)

optimal cutoff value before the initiation of treatment, they could strongly predict the patient outcome. After validation with future trials, they suggested that such parameters, or modified versions of the same, could be used in routine clinical practice and could eventually end up replacing the more invasive methods currently in use for correct prognostication and staging of the cancer. Similar to this, ^{18}F-FDG-PET/CT imaging could be used to assess the global level of involvement in TB, and such studies are highly encouraged (**Figs. 5** and **6**).[48]

Studies[38,49,50] assessing the importance of the different characteristics of TB lesions found in the lung as well as at extrapulmonary sites and the findings seen on ^{18}F-FDG-PET/CT imaging suggested that it could enhance the quality of evaluation, assessment, and management of patients with TB. Malherbe and colleagues[49] examined the MLV, SUVmax, and SUVmean, and the total glycolytic activity, which is MLV × SUVmean, for the lung lesions while quantifying TB lesions.[49] However, they used the conventional quantitative methods of analysis assessing the volume of uptake of the single largest lesion in TB, rather than considering global disease uptake. As mentioned by Salavati and colleagues,[43] the conventional methods that have been used most commonly assess only the disease activity of the largest lesion. The studies conducted on using FDG-PET/CT in TB[4,5,10] have only considered the disease activity of the largest TB lesion in the lung. The largest TB lesion in the lung alone does not accurately represent the complete spectrum of disease activity in the body and can underestimate the functional loss caused by the disease. Hence, it is prudent to consider methods that look at the whole-body disease involvement rather than just the largest lesion.

In short, pretreatment uptake of ^{18}F-FDG by lesions followed by analysis of the uptake during treatment at fixed timeframes, quantifying the changes seen in the lesion uptake after initiation of treatment, and correlating them with clinical findings would help in tailoring the treatment of TB individually. This could go a long way in improving the quality of life, which is significantly affected when different combinations of antituberculous drugs are prescribed in drug-resistant TB by trial-and-error method. Early assessment of the changes with FDG-PET/CT looking at an early detection of change in the disease course could prompt change in patient management, specify therapy, avoid undertreatment or overtreatment, and hence, reduce medication side effects.

SUMMARY

FDG-PET/CT is becoming an important imaging technique for the assessment of patients with TB. This imaging modality mainly contributes to disease detection, assessment of the extent of the disease, and treatment response monitoring in TB. PET/CT continues to play a major role in developing treatment strategies, for instance, MDR-TB cases. One of the main shortcomings of PET/CT is the lack of a standard quantitative technique. The explained global disease assessment technique in this review may overcome the existing shortcomings of the current techniques.

REFERENCES

1. Daley CL. The global fight against tuberculosis. Thorac Surg Clin 2019;29(1):19–25.
2. Chin KL, Sarmiento ME, Norazmi MN, et al. DNA markers for tuberculosis diagnosis. Tuberculosis (Edinb) 2018;113:139–52.
3. Khan PY, Yates TA, Osman M, et al. Transmission of drug-resistant tuberculosis in HIV-endemic settings. Lancet Infect Dis 2019;19(3):e77–88.
4. Johnson DH, Via LE, Kim P, et al. Nuclear imaging: a powerful novel approach for tuberculosis. Nucl Med Biol 2014;41(10):777–84.
5. Wallis RS, Maeurer M, Mwaba P, et al. Tuberculosis—advances in development of new drugs, treatment regimens, host-directed therapies, and biomarkers. Lancet Infect Dis 2016;16(4):e34–46.
6. Sathekge M, Maes A, D'Asseler Y, et al. Nuclear medicine imaging in tuberculosis using commercially available radiopharmaceuticals. Nucl Med Commun 2012;33(6):581–90.
7. Sathekge M, Maes A, Wiele CVD. FDG-PET imaging in HIV infection and tuberculosis. Semin Nucl Med 2013;43(5):349–66.
8. Geadas C, Acuna-Villaorduna C, Mercier G, et al. FDG-PET/CT activity leads to the diagnosis of unsuspected TB: a retrospective study. BMC Res Notes 2018;11(1):464.
9. Maturu VN, Agarwal R, Aggarwal AN, et al. Dual-time point whole-body18F-fluorodeoxyglucose PET/CT imaging in undiagnosed mediastinal lymphadenopathy: a prospective study of 117 patients with sarcoidosis and TB. Chest 2014;146(6):e216–20.
10. Ankrah AO, Glaudemans AWJM, Maes A, et al. Tuberculosis. Semin Nucl Med 2018;48(2):108–30.
11. Ito K, Morooka M, Minamimoto R, et al. Imaging spectrum and pitfalls of (1)(8)F-fluorodeoxyglucose positron emission tomography/computed tomography in patients with tuberculosis. Jpn J Radiol 2013;31(8):511–20.
12. Agarwal KK, Behera A, Kumar R, et al. (18)F-Fluorodeoxyglucose-positron emission tomography/

computed tomography in tuberculosis: spectrum of manifestations. Indian J Nucl Med 2017;32(4): 316–21.

13. Ankrah AO, van der Werf TS, de Vries EFJ, et al. PET/CT imaging of Mycobacterium tuberculosis infection. Clin Transl Imaging 2016;4:131–44.

14. Li Y, Su M, Li F, et al. The value of (1)(8)F-FDG-PET/CT in the differential diagnosis of solitary pulmonary nodules in areas with a high incidence of tuberculosis. Ann Nucl Med 2011;25(10):804–11.

15. Burrill J, Williams CJ, Bain G, et al. Tuberculosis: a radiologic review. Radiographics 2007;27(5): 1255–73.

16. Sakakibara Y, Suzuki Y, Fujie T, et al. Radiopathological features and identification of mycobacterial infections in granulomatous nodules resected from the lung. Respiration 2017;93(4):264–70.

17. Kang F, Wang S, Tian F, et al. Comparing the diagnostic potential of 68Ga-alfatide II and 18F-FDG in differentiating between non-small cell lung cancer and tuberculosis. J Nucl Med 2016;57(5):672–7.

18. Auld SC, Shah NS, Cohen T, et al. Where is tuberculosis transmission happening? Insights from the literature, new tools to study transmission and implications for the elimination of tuberculosis. Respirology 2018;23:807–17. [Epub ahead of print].

19. Geng E, Kreiswirth B, Burzynski J, et al. Clinical and radiographic correlates of primary and reactivation tuberculosis: a molecular epidemiology study. JAMA 2005;293(22):2740–5.

20. Gambhir S, Ravina M, Rangan K, et al. Imaging in extrapulmonary tuberculosis. Int J Infect Dis 2017; 56:237–47.

21. Karunanithi S, Kumar G, Sharma P, et al. Potential role of 18F-2-fluoro-2-deoxy-glucose positron emission tomography/computed tomography imaging in patients presenting with generalized lymphadenopathy. Indian J Nucl Med 2015;30(1):31.

22. Lefebvre N, Argemi X, Meyer N, et al. Clinical usefulness of 18F-FDG PET/CT for initial staging and assessment of treatment efficacy in patients with lymph node tuberculosis. Nucl Med Biol 2017;50:17–24.

23. Micera R, Simoni N, De Liguoro M, et al. The key role of 18F-FDG PET/CT for correct diagnosis, staging, and treatment in a patient with simultaneous NPC and TB lymphadenitis: case report. Tumori 2016; 102(2_suppl):S22–5.

24. Sun Y, Yu H, Ma J, et al. The role of 18F-FDG PET/CT integrated imaging in distinguishing malignant from benign pleural effusion. PLoS One 2016;11(8): e0161764.

25. Akdogan RA, Rakici H, Güngör S, et al. F-18 Fluorodeoxyglucose positron emission tomography/computed tomography findings of isolated gastric tuberculosis mimicking gastric cancer and lymphoma. Euroasian J Hepatogastroenterol 2018; 8(1):93.

26. Yu H-Y, Sheng J-F. Liver tuberculosis presenting as an uncommon cause of pyrexia of unknown origin: positron emission tomography/computed tomography identifies the correct site for biopsy. Med Princ Pract 2014;23(6):577–9.

27. Chen R, Chen Y, Liu L, et al. The role of 18F-FDG PET/CT in the evaluation of peritoneal thickening of undetermined origin. Medicine 2016;95(15):e3023.

28. Rivas-Garcia A, Sarria-Estrada S, Torrents-Odin C, et al. Imaging findings of Pott's disease. Eur Spine J 2013;22(4):567–78.

29. Vorster M, Sathekge MM, Bomanji J. Advances in imaging of tuberculosis: the role of 18F-FDG PET and PET/CT. Curr Opin Pulm Med 2014;20(3): 287–93.

30. Gambhir S, Kumar M, Ravina M, et al. Role of 18F-FDG PET in demonstrating disease burden in patients with tuberculous meningitis. J Neurol Sci 2016;370:196–200.

31. Testempassi E, Kubota K, Morooka M, et al. Constrictive tuberculous pericarditis diagnosed using 18 F-fluorodeoxyglucose positron emission tomography: a report of two cases. Ann Nucl Med 2010;24(5):421–5.

32. Smith I. Mycobacterium tuberculosis pathogenesis and molecular determinants of virulence. Clin Microbiol Rev 2003;16(3):463–96.

33. Eddy J, Khan T, Schembri F. Medical management of drug-sensitive active thoracic tuberculosis: the work-up, radiographic findings and treatment. J Thorac Dis 2018;10(Suppl 28):S3378.

34. Belknap RW. Current medical management of pulmonary tuberculosis. Thorac Surg Clin 2019;29(1): 27–35.

35. Demura Y, Tsuchida T, Uesaka D, et al. Usefulness of 18 F-fluorodeoxyglucose positron emission tomography for diagnosing disease activity and monitoring therapeutic response in patients with pulmonary mycobacteriosis. Eur J Nucl Med Mol Imaging 2009; 36(4):632–9.

36. Martinez V, Castilla-Lievre MA, Guillet-Caruba C, et al. 18F-FDG PET/CT in tuberculosis: an early non-invasive marker of therapeutic response. Int J Tuberc Lung Dis 2012;16(9):1180–5.

37. Chen RY, Dodd LE, Lee M, et al. PET/CT imaging correlates with treatment outcome in patients with multidrug-resistant tuberculosis. Sci Transl Med 2014;6(265):265ra166.

38. Choi J, Jhun B, Hyun S, et al. 18F-Fluorodeoxyglucose positron emission tomography/computed tomography for assessing treatment response of pulmonary multidrug-resistant tuberculosis. J Clin Med 2018;7(12):559.

39. Houshmand S, Salavati A, Hess S, et al. An update on novel quantitative techniques in the context of evolving whole-body PET imaging. PET Clin 2015; 10(1):45–58.

40. Sadeghi R, Harsini S, Qodsi Rad MA, et al. Prognostic significance of fluorine-18 fluorodeoxyglucose positron emission tomography in anal squamous cell carcinoma: a systematic review and a meta-analysis. Contrast Media Mol Imaging 2018;2018:9760492.

41. Martens RM, Noij DP, Ali M, et al. Functional imaging early during (chemo)radiotherapy for response prediction in head and neck squamous cell carcinoma; a systematic review. Oral Oncol 2019;88: 75–83.

42. Brinkman M, Jentjens S, Boone K, et al. Evaluation of the most commonly used (semi-)quantitative parameters of 18F-FDG PET/CT to detect malignant transformation of neurofibromas in neurofibromatosis type 1. Nucl Med Commun 2018;39(11):961–8.

43. Salavati A, Duan F, Snyder BS, et al. Optimal FDG PET/CT volumetric parameters for risk stratification in patients with locally advanced non-small cell lung cancer: results from the ACRIN 6668/RTOG 0235 trial. Eur J Nucl Med Mol Imaging 2017; 44(12):1969–83.

44. Li Q, Zhang J, Cheng W, et al. Prognostic value of maximum standard uptake value, metabolic tumor volume, and total lesion glycolysis of positron emission tomography/computed tomography in patients with nasopharyngeal carcinoma: a systematic review and meta-analysis. Medicine (Baltimore) 2017;96(37):e8084.

45. Zhu D, Wang L, Zhang H, et al. Prognostic value of 18F-FDG-PET/CT parameters in patients with pancreatic carcinoma: a systematic review and meta-analysis. Medicine (Baltimore) 2017;96(33): e7813.

46. Huang Y, Feng M, He Q, et al. Prognostic value of pretreatment 18F-FDG PET-CT for nasopharyngeal carcinoma patients. Medicine (Baltimore) 2017; 96(17):e6721.

47. Lin J, Xie G, Liao G, et al. Prognostic value of 18F-FDG-PET/CT in patients with nasopharyngeal carcinoma: a systematic review and meta-analysis. Oncotarget 2017;8(20):33884–96.

48. Alavi A, Hess S, Werner TJ, et al. An update on the unparalleled impact of FDG-PET imaging on the day-to-day practice of medicine with emphasis on management of infectious/inflammatory disorders. Eur J Nucl Med Mol Imaging 2020 Jan;47(1):18–27.

49. Malherbe ST, Dupont P, Kant I, et al. A semi-automatic technique to quantify complex tuberculous lung lesions on 18 F-fluorodeoxyglucose positron emission tomography/computerised tomography images. EJNMMI Res 2018;8(1):55.

50. Martin C, Castaigne C, Vierasu I, et al. Prospective serial FDG PET/CT during treatment of extrapulmonary tuberculosis in HIV-infected patients: an exploratory study. Clin Nucl Med 2018;43(9):635–40.

Printed and bound by CPI Group (UK) Ltd, Croydon, CR0 4YY

08/06/2025

01896875-0014